Autism and Child Psychopathology Series

Series Editor

Johnny L. Matson, Baton Rouge, LA, USA

Brief Overview

The purpose of this series is to advance knowledge in the broad multidisciplinary fields of autism and various forms of psychopathology (e.g., anxiety and depression). Volumes synthesize research on a range of rapidly expanding topics on assessment, treatment, and etiology.

Description

The **Autism and Child Psychopathology Series** explores a wide range of research and professional methods, procedures, and theories used to enhance positive development and outcomes across the lifespan. Developments in education, medicine, psychology, and applied behavior analysis as well as child and adolescent development across home, school, hospital, and community settings are the focus of this series. Series volumes are both authored and edited, and they provide critical reviews of evidence-based methods. As such, these books serve as a critical reference source for researchers and professionals who deal with developmental disorders and disabilities, most notably autism, intellectual disabilities, challenging behaviors, anxiety, depression, ADHD, developmental coordination disorder, communication disorders, and other common childhood problems. The series addresses important mental health and development difficulties that children and youth, their caregivers, and the professionals who treat them must face. Each volume in the series provides an analysis of methods and procedures that may assist in effectively treating these developmental problems.

Jeff Sigafoos • Giulio E. Lancioni
Mark F. O'Reilly

Communication Strategies for People with Severe Disabilities

Springer

Jeff Sigafoos
School of Education
Victoria University of Wellington
Wellington, New Zealand

Giulio E. Lancioni
Lega F. D'Oro Research Center
Osimo (AN), Italy

Mark F. O'Reilly
Department of Special Education
The University of Texas at Austin
Austin, TX, USA

ISSN 2192-922X ISSN 2192-9238 (electronic)
Autism and Child Psychopathology Series
ISBN 978-3-031-83806-4 ISBN 978-3-031-83807-1 (eBook)
https://doi.org/10.1007/978-3-031-83807-1

This Springer imprint is published by the registered company Springer Nature Switzerland AG
The registered company address is: Gewerbestrasse 11, 6330 Cham, Switzerland

Preface

The acquisition of speech and language is an impressive accomplishment that most children achieve around 3–4 years of age. However, not all children develop spoken language to anywhere near the degree that would be needed for effective communication. Indeed, a significant percentage of children fail to develop any appreciable amount of spoken language ability. Individuals can also develop communication impairment later in life due to an acquired condition.

In the absence of speech, what strategies can people with severe disabilities use to communicate? This book addresses this question by describing alternatives to speech that have enabled individuals with severe disability to communicate more effectively using socially and age-appropriate strategies. The strategies considered in this book are the means or modes by which a person could express their wants and needs, make comments, exchange information, and more generally participate in social-communicative exchanges with family, friends, teachers, employers, and other people in their wider community.

The separate chapters in this book are each devoted to the use of a distinct communication strategy, specifically: prelinguistic communication (Chap. 3), natural gestures (Chap. 4), manual signing (Chap. 5), tangible symbols (Chap. 6), picture exchange (Chap. 7), and speech-generating devices (Chap. 8). Subsequent chapters consider solutions for individuals with additional sensory and motor impairments (Chap. 9) and receptive language difficulties (Chap. 10).

These chapters review key research studies related to the use of each respective strategy. We consider each strategy's pros and cons and evaluate interventions for teaching effective use of each strategy. The aim is to review studies that illustrate for practitioners the successful application of instructional procedures for teaching functional use of specific communication strategies.

Selecting a viable communication strategy and using it successfully requires an understanding of the cognitive, learning, and behavioral characteristics associated with severe disability (Chap. 1). It is also important to understand the general nature of communication functioning of people with severe disabilities and strategies for assessing their communication functioning (Chap. 2).

Overall, the content covered in the ten chapters of this book will hopefully be of value to practitioners and researchers across the range of disciplines that are relevant to supporting the communication development of individuals with severe disabilities, such as applied behavior analysis, augmentative and alternative communication, communication disorders, rehabilitation engineering, special education, and speech-language pathology.

Wellington, New Zealand Jeff Sigafoos
Osimo, Italy Giulio E. Lancioni
Austin, TX, USA Mark F. O'Reilly

Contents

About the Authors

Jeff Sigafoos is a professor in the School of Education at Victoria University of Wellington. He undertakes research on the application of systematic instructional procedures for teaching adaptive skills to children and adults with severe disabilities, including teaching communication skills to nonverbal individuals with developmental disabilities.

Giulio E. Lancioni is the Director of the Lega F. D'Oro Research Center in Osimo, Italy. He specializes in the use of assistive technology interventions to enhance the adaptive behavior functioning of people with severe, profound, and multiple disabilities.

Mark F. O'Reilly is the Melissa Elizabeth Stuart Centennial Professor in the Department of Special Education at the University of Texas at Austin. His research focuses on teaching adaptive skills to individuals with severe disabilities and on the assessment and treatment of challenging behavior of individuals with autism and other developmental disabilities.

Chapter 1
Describing Severe Disability

Defining and Describing Severe Disability

The term severe disability references a broad category that encompasses a number of more specific conditions. Primarily, the category encompasses people with substantial cognitive and adaptive functioning limitations associated with intellectual disability, autism spectrum disorder, and/or cerebral palsy (American Psychiatric Association, 2013; Haslan, 2017; Vitrikas et al., 2020). However, the term could also be applied to some individuals with traumatic brain injury and certain neurological conditions, such as Alzheimer's disease, amyotrophic lateral sclerosis, and other motor neuron diseases (Lamptey et al., 2022; Tenovuo et al., 2021).

Within each of these specific conditions, the severity of the impairment can vary from relatively mild to more severe/profound and change over time. Thus, not all individuals with autism and/or intellectual disability, for example, would necessarily have a severe disability. In fact, many, if not most, individuals with autism or intellectual disability present with a relatively mild-to-moderate degree of disability. Still, a significant percentage of people with one or more of the above types of disability conditions will present with, or progress to, severe levels of impairment. Table 1.1 provides definitions and classification approaches for the most prevalent disability conditions associated with impaired cognitive and adaptive behavior functioning.

The determination of whether or not someone should be described as having a severe disability, as opposed to say a more mild-to-moderate degree of disability, therefore depends on the nature and extent of their impairments. As noted by Reichle (1997), severe disability generally refers to situations where an individual experiences significant impairment in one or more major areas of cognitive and/or adaptive behavior functioning. A severe disability may also stem from greatly impaired physical/motor or sensory impairment, such as when a person is quadriplegic and confined to a wheelchair or is both deaf and blind. Impairment in one or more of

J. Sigafoos et al., *Communication Strategies for People with Severe Disabilities*, Autism and Child Psychopathology Series,
https://doi.org/10.1007/978-3-031-83807-1_1

Table 1.1 Definition and classification of conditions associated with impaired cognitive and adaptive behavior functioning

Condition	Definition	Classification of severity	Source
Autism spectrum disorder	A neurodevelopmental disorder characterized by "persistent impairment in social communication and social interaction" and "restricted, repetitive patterns of behavior, interests, or activities" that arise in "early developmental period"	Three levels of severity have been proposed depending on degree of communication and social skills deficits and the extent to which restricted/ repetitive behaviors interfere with functioning	American Psychiatric Association (2013, p. 50)
Cerebral palsy	A group of permanent non-progressive physical disabilities due to injury to the developing brain that affects movement, posture, and balance	Can range from mild to severe depending on nature of disorder (spasticity or ataxia) and which limbs are involved (diplegia versus quadriplegia)	Vitrikas et al. (2020)
Intellectual disability	Significantly sub-average general intellectual functioning and adaptive behavior deficits evident during the developmental period	Level of severity (i.e., mild, moderate, severe, and profound) are based on degree of intellectual and adaptive behavior impairments	American Psychiatric Association (2013)
Traumatic brain injury	Brain damage caused by external forces, such as direct impact	Severity classified as mild, moderate, or severe depending on motor control and verbal responding	Silver et al. (2019)
Alzheimer's disease	A neurodegenerative disorder affecting brain cells and resulting in the loss of cognitive functions (e.g., memory) and adaptive skills	Classified as preclinical, mild, moderate, or severe depending on degree of memory loss, disorientation, concentration, mood, impulse control, loss of self-care and adaptive skills, and reading, writing, and speaking difficulties	Breijyeh and Karaman (2020)
Motor neuron diseases	Inherited or acquired group of diseases that result in the loss of motor neurons, which impacts motor control and leads to muscle wasting and weakness, spasticity, and hyperreflexia	The nature and severity of motor impairment can vary and decrease over time. More severe cases are associated with complete loss of ambulation, very limited voluntary motor control, loss of speech, and shortened life	Jorgensen et al. (2020)

these major functioning domains is considered to represent a severe disability if the impairments have significant and long-term negative impacts on the person's learning, development, independence, life opportunities, and overall quality of life.

With respect to overall quality of life, Ncube et al. (2018) found that children with severe disabilities were rated as having a significantly lower quality of life compared to typically developing children. Quality of life was lowest for older children who had more limited levels of adaptive behavior and higher levels of problem behavior. Similar findings have been reported in numerous other studies (Luitwieler et al., 2021). Collectively, these findings highlight the potential benefits on quality of life from effective interventions aimed at decreasing problem behavior and increasing adaptive skills, including development of the person's communication skills. Indeed, Sigafoos et al. (2010) argued that improved quality of life through adaptive skills training, including teaching communication skills, should be a major objective in educational and therapy programs for persons with severe disabilities.

Prevalence

Intellectual Disability

Global prevalence estimates for intellectual disability consistently cite a figure of around 1% or 10 per 1000 (Maulik et al., 2011). However, this figure pertains to the full age range (children, adolescents, and adults) as well as all severity levels (i.e., mild, moderate, and severe/profound). Given that most cases of intellectual disability are classified as mild to moderate, the prevalence of severe intellectual disability is much lower than the commonly cited 1% figure. Prevalence estimates also tend to be higher for child versus adult samples. However, severe intellectual disability remains a significant and prevalent concern. Considering just children with severe intellectual disability (IQ < 50), van Bakel et al. (2013) found prevalence figures ranging from 3.0 (in France) to 5.1 (in Iceland) per 1000 or from 0.3 to 0.51%. The American Psychiatric Association (2013) published a higher prevalence figure (6 per 1000 or 0.6%) for severe intellectual disability. These varying estimates have been attributed in part to varying diagnostic and case ascertainment methods across countries (van Bakel et al., 2013). Based on these figures, it would seem reasonable to conclude that the prevalence of severe intellectual disability is somewhere in the range of about 0.3–0.6% or 3–6 per 1000.

Autism Spectrum Disorder

Prevalence estimates for autism spectrum disorder tend to mirror those reported for intellectual disability. That is, the overall average global prevalence estimate for autism spectrum disorder has also been reported to be about 1% or 10 per 1000 (Zeidan et al., 2022). And, as for intellectual disability, the distribution of severity levels is skewed toward the milder end of the spectrum. The prevalence of more severe/profound autism—characterized by major deficits in both intellectual (IQ < 50) and adaptive behavior functioning—was estimated at 4.6 per 1000

(0.46%) among a large sample (n = 20,135) of 8-year-old children (Hughes et al., 2023). About 33% of people with autism also meet the diagnostic criteria for intellectual disability (Zeidan et al., 2022). Clarke et al. (2024) used the term profound autism to refer to individuals with autism and co-occurring severe intellectual disability (IQ < 50). They noted that such individuals also tend to have limited or no spoken language, and require high levels of care. Profound autism was estimated to make up about 20% of all autism cases. Thus, in a representative sample of autistic individuals, one could expect that a "sizeable minority" of these people would have profound autism characterized by severe intellectual disability, limited or no speech, and requiring extremely high levels of care (Clarke et al., 2024, p. 10).

Cerebral Palsy

Prevalence figures for cerebral palsy range from about 1.6 to 3.1 per 1000 (Christensen et al., 2014; Maenner et al., 2016; McIntyre et al., 2022; Oskoui et al., 2013; van Gorp et al., 2020). However, estimates vary markedly in line with a country's economic level. Specifically, in a study covering 27 countries, McIntyre et al. (2022) reported a prevalence figure of 3.4 per 1000 (0.34%) in low- to middle-income countries, but a much lower figure (1.5 per 1000 or 0.15%) in high-income countries. Interestingly, McIntyre et al. also found evidence for there being a decreasing trend in the prevalence of cerebral palsy in high-income countries. Cerebral palsy can vary from mild to severe depending on the type and degree of motoric and postural impairment. Some people with cerebral palsy experience relatively mild involuntary muscle contractions (i.e., spasticity) or writhing movements (athetosis), whereas other people experience more severe muscle contractions affecting all four limbs (i.e., spastic quadriplegia), which can result in the person being "almost completely physically incapacitated" (Steppe-Jones et al., 2014, p. 492). In addition, intellectual disability, autism, and epilepsy are common co-occurring conditions among people with cerebral palsy. For example, surveys report that about 41.3% of children with cerebral palsy present with moderate-to-severe intellectual disability, 6.9–8.7% with autism, and 30.5–41% with epilepsy (Christensen et al., 2014; Delobel-Ayoub et al., 2017; Gabis et al., 2015).

Traumatic Brain Injury

Traumatic brain injuries are estimated to occur in approximately 12% of adults (Frost et al., 2013). For many of these individuals, their brain injury would have occurred during childhood or adolescence (McKinlay et al., 2008). However, the percentage of adults who have experienced a severe traumatic brain injury (i.e., with loss of consciousness) is much lower at about 2.6% (Corrigan et al., 2018). This 2.6% figure makes traumatic brain injury more prevalent than severe intellectual disability, autism spectrum disorder, or cerebral palsy. The relatively high prevalence of severe traumatic brain injury highlights a need for better preventative efforts as well as effective interventions to ameliorate and/or compensate for any lingering functioning limitations (Silver et al., 2019).

Alzheimer's Disease

A similar intervention call is relevant to the estimated 25 million people worldwide suffering from dementia, most of whom have Alzheimer's disease (Breijyeh & Karaman, 2020; Qui et al., 2009). Alzheimer's and related dementias are progressive and mainly affect the aged. Predictably then, severe cases—resulting in substantial functioning limitations, including communication impairment—are likely to increase in countries with aging populations.

Motor Neuron Diseases

Another group who are likely to become progressively less capable over time are the estimated 300+ thousand people across the globe who are living with a motor neuron (nerve cell) disease, such as amyotrophic lateral sclerosis or spinal muscular atrophy. This class of diseases affects the nerve cells that regulate upper and/or lower body muscles (Jorgensen et al., 2020). The overall prevalence of such diseases is relatively rare (about 4–5 per 100,000) with amyotrophic lateral sclerosis being the most prevalent type of motor neuron disease, accounting for 85% of cases (Logroscino et al., 2018). Motor neuron diseases nearly always lead eventually to severe functioning limitations and reduced life expectancy. Amyotrophic lateral sclerosis, for example, tends to be fatal within 20–48 months from the onset of symptoms, with about 70% of patients dying within 36 months of symptom onset (Bianchi et al., 2022).

Cognitive Impairments

It is generally the case that multiple areas of cognitive functioning are significantly impaired in people with severe disability. In the cognitive domain, as mentioned previously, a classification of severe to profound intellectual ability is generally applied to situations in which the person has scored extremely low (IQ < 50) on an appropriately administered, individualized intelligence test. IQ scores in this range indicate major deficits in intellectual ability and predict limited general knowledge as well as reduced capacity for reasoning, problem solving, and analytic thinking. Many such individuals will also have impaired working (short-term) memory, spatial recognition difficulties, and a limited understanding of the concept of time (O'Reilly & Carr, 2016). Literacy and numeracy skills are also likely to be severely limited in most instances of severe/profound intellectual disability (Hunt et al., 2020). Similar cognitive problems are found among some individuals with profound autism and cerebral palsy (Bhat, 2021; Stadskleiv, 2020).

Cognitive impairments are also associated with traumatic brain injury. Skandsen et al. (2010), for example, assessed the cognitive abilities of 61 traumatic brain injury patients. These patients ranged from 15 to 65 years of age and had suffered a moderate-to-severe brain injury. The results showed that traumatic brain injury patients had significant deficits with respect to information processing, speech, and verbal memory compared to 47 controls who had not suffered any brain injuries. Interestingly, 50% of the patients with moderate brain injury and 33% of patients who had suffered a severe brain injury showed normal levels of cognitive functioning at an assessment conducted 3 months after the injury. Thus, long-term cognitive impairment is not inevitable even in cases of severe traumatic brain injury.

Cognitive impairments have also been well document in people with Alzheimer's disease (Weiner & Lipton, 2012). Impairments can occur across several cognitive functions (e.g., remembering, reasoning, decision-making, concentration, and learning). The degree of impairment can range from mild to severe. In severe cases, patients appear to have little to no capacity to perform basic executive functions, such as making plans, following instructions, staying focused to complete tasks, or managing their emotions and impulses (Voisin & Vellas, 2009).

With respect to the motor neuron diseases, Lillo and Hodges (2010) reviewed literature on the cognitive abilities of people with motor neuron diseases. They concluded that cognitive impairment is predictive of more rapid disease progression and shortened life. However, cognitive decline did not occur in most such patients and when it did the degree of cognitive decline was often relatively mild.

Adaptive Behavior Deficits

Adaptive behavior is an important psychological construct. Understanding this construct is critical for understanding the nature and degree of functioning impairments experienced by people with the types of developmental and acquired disabilities described in Table 1.1. Information about a person's adaptive behavior functioning is used for diagnosis and classification purposes and for making educational and treatment decisions, such as prioritizing treatment goals and selecting intervention strategies.

Tassé (2021) noted that adaptive behavior is "a broad construct that encompasses practical skills...social skills... and conceptual skills..." (p. 1). Practical skills encompass the actions that are needed to complete self-care routines (e.g., dressing, toileting, and washing). More generally, practical skills are those everyday behaviors that are required in order to be able to function with some degree of independence across a range of domestic, school, community, and vocational/employment settings (e.g., meal preparation, home cleaning and maintenance, shopping, pedestrian safety skills, and job performance). Social skills include emotional regulation, interacting with others appropriately, and following social conventions. Conceptual skills include functional academics (e.g., sight word reading), time and money management, and self-direction, which involves decision-making and self-initiation.

Adaptive skills are typically organized into one of several distinct domains of functioning. For example, the third edition of the Vineland Adaptive Behavior Scales (Sparrow et al., 2016)—a widely used measures of adaptive behavior functioning—delineates five functioning domains: (a) communication, (b) daily living, (c) socialization, (d) motor skills, and (e) maladaptive behavior. Each of these domains is further divided into subdomains, which list specific adaptive skills. The daily living skills domain, for example, includes personal skills (e.g., feeds self with a spoon), domestic skills (e.g., prepares a simple snack or meal), and community skills (e.g., looks both ways when crossing streets or roads). The socialization domain, in contrast, consists of the following three subdomains: (a) interpersonal relationships (e.g., smiles in response to praise, imitates facial expressions, and uses actions or words to show happiness or concern), (b) play and leisure (e.g., plays near another child, shares toys, and follows rules in games), and (c) coping skills (e.g., seeks comfort from parents when hurt, is polite when asking for something, and accepts helpful suggestions).

The communication domain of adaptive behavior functioning encompasses speech and language ability as well as the extent to which other expressive communication skills (e.g., manual signing and natural gestures) have developed. Receptive language and written communication are also aspects or subdomains within the broader area of communication. Chap. 2 describes the communication domain more fully and considers the assessment of communicative functioning in people with severe disabilities.

People with severe disability experience substantial deficits across multiple adaptive behavior functioning domains. Matson et al. (1998), for example, documented significant deficits across multiple adaptive functioning domains, including very limited social skills, in a sample of 892 children and adults with diagnoses of severe-to-profound intellectual disability. Using the Vineland Adaptive Behavior Scales, Fenton et al. (2003) also found significant deficits across multiple functioning domains in samples of children (21–108 months of age) with autism and moderate-to-severe disability (n = 23) and children with moderate-to-severe disability, but not autism (n = 27). The adaptive behavior profiles were similar for both groups of children and characterized by equally large deficits across the communication, daily living, and socialization domains.

Similar data have been reported in relation to traumatic brain injury and motor neuron diseases (Anderson et al., 2012; Simmons, 2013). Anderson et al., for example, found that children who had suffered a severe traumatic brain injury had behavioral and social skill impairments as well as major problems with executive functioning, and greatly reduced quality of life when assessed 6 months after the injury. The same range and degree of impairment and reduction of quality of life were not found in children who had suffered more mild brain injuries. In cases of severe Alzheimer's disease, basic self-care and communication ability—both expressive and receptive communication—can be completely lost, making the person totally dependent on others. In addition, as the disease progressively worsens, a range of disturbing personality changes may emerge, sometimes including delusions, hallucinations, extreme agitation, and/or aggression (Voisin & Vellas, 2009).

Learning and Behavioral Characteristics

People with severe disabilities often exhibit certain anomalous learning and behavioral characteristics that can make efforts to teach them more difficult. Sigafoos and colleagues (Sigafoos et al., 2020, 2021) summarized literature on some of the more common learning and behavioral characteristics that have been documented among people with severe disability. The often cited learning and behavioral characteristics associated with severe disability include biased response patterns, outer-directedness, motivational and attentional problems, and problem behavior.

Biased Response Patterns

Some people with severe disability adopt biased or random response patterns that are counter-productive for learning and problem solving (Diamond, 2018). For example, in a learning task that requires selecting symbols from an array of two or more options (e.g., point to X versus point to Y), learners with severe disabilities might fall into a pattern of always selecting whatever picture is closest, or on the right, or on the left, etc.—a strategy known as position-biased responding. Others might gravitate toward whatever picture is bigger or more colorful (item-biased responding) or respond by simply alternating from one option to the other. Still others might respond in a seemingly random pattern. These types of response patterns could make it more difficult to teach the person more complex discrimination skills that are often required for functional communication, such as learning to select the correct communication symbol to indicate *YES* versus *NO*.

Outer-Directedness

Another learning characteristic that has been frequently reported among individuals with severe disabilities is seeking cues and help from others when faced with a relatively difficult task or problem to solve (Bybee & Zigler, 1998). For example, when asked to solve a puzzle, children with intellectual disability will often seek cues and help from any adult present (Kasari & Freeman, 2001). This phenomenon is known as outer-directedness. MacMillan and Cauffiel (1977) noted that "outerdirectedness represents a motivational style of problem solving in which the child uses external cues rather than relying on his own cognitive resources" (p. 643). The tendency toward outer-directedness indicates that individuals with intellectual disability can recognize and act on the often subtle and inadvertent cues provided by others, such as when a teacher momentarily glances at the correct item in a two-choice matching task. The ability to read external subtle cues and then use these cues to solve problems could be seen as showing a rather impressive degree of social awareness. It is also a form of developmentally appropriate social referencing that is commonly observed in young children without disabilities. However, over-reliance on such cues as a problem-solving strategy is ultimately counterproductive because it limits independence.

Motivational Problems

People with severe disabilities have also been described as lacking motivation (Hickson & Khemka, 2013), but this a somewhat contentious issue. Research examining the extent to which there are motivational deficits in people with intellectual disability, for example, has produced mixed results (Cuskelly & Gilmore, 2014). Still, it does appear that people with severe disabilities often show little or no initiation with respect to functional activities and social–communication interactions. In addition, such individuals may give up easily, especially when they have experienced some initial failure or are confronted with a relatively new or more difficult task. These behavior patterns could signal some type of motivational problem, but might also be related to environmental conditions and experiences (Cuskelly & Gilmore, 2014). For example, it is possible that a learner with severe disability may remain passive or attempt to escape and avoid learning situations due to repeated past failure, ineffective types and schedules of reinforcement, and limited understanding of task requirements. In addition, motivation may wane if participation requires physical and/or cognitive efforts that are beyond the person's present capabilities (Sigafoos et al., 2020, pp. 179–180). It has long been noted that success in teaching people with severe disabilities to use the various types of communication strategies described in later chapters of this book will likely depend to some extent on creating, capturing, boosting, and maintaining their motivation to communicate (Koegel & Koegel, 1995).

Attentional Problems

Attentional problems have also been highlighted as a potential barrier to effective learning for people with severe disabilities (Follmer, 2018). The degree of attentional problems is often of sufficient magnitude that the person may receive a diagnosis of attention-deficit hyperactivity disorder (Neece et al., 2011). Attentional problems may manifest as a limited attention span, use of inefficient problem-solving strategies, failure to attend to or comprehend task instructions before responding, and/or failure to attend to the relevant aspects of instructional stimuli. This latter pattern has been referred to as selective attention or stimulus over-selectivity (Lovaas et al., 1979). Such problems could indicate underlying cognitive processing deficits, but might also stem from ineffective teaching and/or motivational issues, such as the person not being interested in the materials or the outcome of a task or activity. It is likely that the different communication strategies covered in Chaps. 3–10 of this book have varying types and degrees of attentional demands, which may influence strategy implementation for any given individual. Fortunately, data indicate that attentional problems can be addressed by directly teaching specific attending skills (Isaksen & Holth, 2009; Plavnick, 2012).

Problem Behavior

Problem behaviors, such as aggression, self-injury, property destruction, and extreme tantrums, are frequently cited in the educational and psychological literature pertaining to people with various conditions, including people with severe disabilities (Cividini-Motta et al., 2017). Aggression and self-injury are particularly prevalent among individuals with severe intellectual disability and autism spectrum disorder. Based on a review of 20 prevalence studies, Simó-Pinatella et al. (2019) found that problematic forms of behavior (mainly aggression and self-injury) were of concern in 48–60% of children with intellectual disability and in up to 90% of children with autism spectrum disorder. These types of problem behavior can lead to serious injury and damage and reduce overall quality of life. Even mildly disruptive behaviors, such as verbal outbursts and stereotyped mannerisms, can interfere with efforts to teach adaptive skills, which may in turn limit the person's ability to participate more fully and independently in home, school, work, and community environments.

Researchers exploring the causes of problem behavior in people with severe disabilities have discovered that these acts often have a learned component and serve an operant function or purpose for the individual (Iwata et al., 1994). Specifically, data indicate that problem behaviors are often maintained by the reinforcing consequences provided by others, such as attention, access to preferred stimuli, or allowing the person to escape from difficult tasks. Problem behavior maintained by these types of reinforcing consequences has been conceptualized as forms of communication related to the pragmatic functions of requesting and rejecting (Durand & Moskowitz, 2019). In line with this conceptualization, a large number of studies have shown that problem behavior can be effectively treated by teaching functional communication, such as teaching the person to request attention or request help with difficult tasks. For these types of interventions, the person with severe disability might be taught to communicate using one or more of the strategies covered in Chaps. 3–10 of this book.

Summary and Conclusion

Severe disabilities are characterized by significant cognitive and/or adaptive functioning impairments. People with severe cognitive and/or adaptive functioning impairments can be found among developmental disability populations, such as people with autism spectrum disorder, cerebral palsy, and intellectual disability. Some people with acquired conditions (e.g., severe traumatic brain injury) and diseases (e.g., motor neuron diseases) can also have severely impaired cognitive and/or adaptive behavior functioning. Severe cognitive and adaptive functioning impairments are likely to make teaching and habilitation efforts, including communication intervention, more difficult. It is also reasonable to hypothesize that implementation of the communication strategies reviewed in Chaps. 3–10 of this book will be more successful when accommodations related to an individual's unique learning and behavioral characteristics are integrated into the overall intervention process.

References

American Psychiatric Association. (2013). *Diagnostic and statistical manual of mental disorders* (5th ed. DSM-5™). American Psychiatric Publishing.

Anderson, V., Le Brocque, R., Iselin, G., Eren, S., Dob, R., Davern, T. J., McKinlay, L., & Kenardy, J. (2012). Adaptive ability behavior and quality of life pre and posttraumatic brain injury in childhood. *Disability & Rehabilitation, 34*(19), 1639–1647. https://doi.org/10.3109/09638288.2012.656789

Bhat, A. N. (2021). Motor impairment increases in children with autism spectrum disorder as a function of social communication, cognitive and functional impairment, repetitive behavior severity, and comorbid diagnosis: A SPARK study report. *Autism Research, 14*(1), 202–219. https://doi.org/10.1002/aur.2453

Bianchi, E., Pupillo, E., De Feudis, A., Enia, G., Vitelli, E., & Beghi, E. (2022). Trends in survival of ALS from a population-based registry. *Amyotrophic Lateral Sclerosis and Frontotemporal Degeneration, 23*(5–6), 344–352. https://doi.org/10.1080/21678421.2021.2004167

Breijyeh, Z., & Karaman, R. (2020). Comprehensive review on Alzheimer's disease: Causes and treatment. *Molecules, 25*(24), 5789. https://doi.org/10.3390/molecules25245789

Bybee, J., & Zigler, E. (1998). Outer-directedness in individuals with and without mental retardation: A review. In J. Burack, R. Hodapp, & E. Zigler (Eds.), *Handbook of mental retardation and development* (pp. 434–461). Cambridge Univerity Press.

Christensen, D., Van Naarden Braun, K., Doemberg, N. S., Maenner, M. J., Arneson, C. L., Durkin, M. S., Benedict, R. E., Kirby, R. S., Wingate, M. S., Fitzgerald, R., & Yeargin-Allsopp, M. (2014). Prevalence of cerebral palsy, co-occurring autism spectrum disorders, and motor functioning—Autism and developmental disabilities monitoring network, USA, 2008. *Developmental Medicine and Child Neurology, 56*, 59–65. https://doi.org/10.1111/dmcn.12268

Cividini-Motta, C., Bloom, S. E., & Campos, C. (2017). Challenging behavior. In J. L. Matson (Ed.), *Handbook of social behavior and skills in children* (pp. 19–45). Springer. https://doi.org/10.1007/978-3-319-64592-6_3

Clarke, E. B., McCauley, J. B., Lutz, A., Gotelli, M., Sheinkopf, S. J., & Lord, C. (2024). Understanding profound autism: Implications for stigma and supports. *Frontiers in Psychiatry, 15*, 1287096. https://doi.org/10.3389/fpsyt.2024.1287096

Corrigan, J. D., Yang, J., Singichetti, B., Manchester, K., & Bogner, J. (2018). Lifetime prevalence of traumatic brain injury with loss of consciousness. *Injury Prevention, 24*(6), 369–404. https://doi.org/10.1136/injuryprev-2017-042371

Cuskelly, M., & Gilmore, L. (2014). Motivation in children with intellectual disabilities. *Research and Practice in Intellectual and Developmental Disabilities, 1*(1), 51–59. https://doi.org/10.1080/23297018.2014.906051

Delobel-Ayoub, M., Klapouszczak, D., van Bakel, M. M. E., Horridge, K., Sigurdardottir, S., Himmelmann, K., & Arnaud, C. (2017). Prevalence and characteristics of autism spectrum disorders in children with cerebral palsy. *Developmental Medicine and Child Neurology, 59*, 738–742. https://doi.org/10.1111/dmcn.13436

Diamond, L. L. (2018). Problem solving using visual support for young children with autism. *Intervention in School and Clinic, 54*(2), 106–110. https://doi.org/10.1177/1053451218765234

Durand, V. M., & Moskowitz, L. J. (2019). The link between problem behavior and communication impairment in persons with developmental disabilities. *Current Developmental Disorders Reports, 6*(3), 138–144. https://doi.org/10.1007/s40474-019-00172-y

Fenton, G., D'Ardia, C., Valente, D., Del Vecchio, I., Fabrizi, A., & Bernabei, P. (2003). Vineland adaptive behavior profiles in children with autism and moderate to severe developmental delay. *Autism, 7*(3), 269–287. https://doi.org/10.1177/1362361303007003004

Follmer, D. J. (2018). Executive function and reading comprehension: A meta-analytic review. *Educational Psychologist, 53*(1), 42–60. https://doi.org/10.1080/00461520.2017.1309295

Frost, R. B., Farrer, T. J., Primosch, M., & Hedges, D. W. (2013). Prevalence of traumatic brain injury in the general adult population: A meta-analysis. *Neuroepidemiology, 40*(3), 154–159. https://doi.org/10.1159/000343275

Gabis, L. V., Tsubary, N. M., Leon, O., Ashkenasi, A., & Shefer, S. (2015). Assessment of abilities and comorbidities in children with cerebral palsy. *Journal of Child Neurology, 30*, 1640–1645. https://doi.org/10.1177/0883073815576792

Haslan, C. (2017). Applications of errorless learning in child rehabilitation. In C. Haslan & R. P. C. Kessels (Eds.), *Errorless learning in neuropsychological rehabilitation: Mechanisms, efficacy and application* (pp. 43–57). Routledge. https://doi.org/10.4324/9781315660738

Hickson, L., & Khemka, I. (2013). Problem solving and decision making. In M. L. Wehmeyer (Ed.), *Oxford handbook of positive psychology and disability* (pp. 198–225). Oxford University Press.

Hughes, M. M., Shaw, K. A., DiRienzo, M., Durkin, M. S., Esler, A., Hall-Lande, J., Wiggins, L., Zahorodny, W., Singer, A., & Maenner, M. J. (2023). The prevalence and characteristics of children with profound autism, 15 sites, United States, 2000-2016. *Public Health Reports, 138*(6), 971–980. https://doi.org/10.1177/00333549231163551

Hunt, P., Kozleski, E., Lee, J., Mortier, K., Fleming, D., Hicks, T., Balasubramanian, L., Leu, G., Bross, L. A., Munandar, V., Dunlap, K., Stepaniuk, I., Aramburo, C., & Oh, Y. (2020). Implementing comprehensive literacy instruction for students with severe disabilities in general education classrooms. *Exceptional Children, 86*(3), 330–347. https://doi.org/10.1177/0014402919880156

Isaksen, J., & Holth, P. (2009). An operant approach to teaching joint attention skills to children with autism. *Behavioral Interventions, 24*(4), 215–236. https://doi.org/10.1002/bin.292

Iwata, B., Pace, G., Dorsey, M., Zarcone, J., Vollmer, T., Smith, R., Rodgers, T., Lerman, D., Shore, B., Mazaleski, J., Goh, H., Cowdery, G., Kalsher, M., McCosh, K., & Willis, K. (1994). The functions of self-injurious behavior: An experimental-epidemiological analysis. *Journal of Applied Behavior Analysis, 27*(2), 215–240. https://doi.org/10.1901/jaba.1994.27-215

Jorgensen, S., Lau, M., & Arnold, W. D. (2020). Motor neuron diseases. In D. X. Cifu (Ed.), *Braddom's physical medicine and rehabilitation* (6th ed., pp. 820–841.e5). Elsevier. https://doi.org/10.1016/C2017-0-03586-3

Kasari, C., & Freeman, S. F. N. (2001). Task-related social behavior in children with down syndrome. *American Journal on Mental Retardation, 106*(3), 253–264. https://doi.org/10.1352/0895-8017(2001)106<0253:TRSBIC>2.0.CO;2

Koegel, L. K., & Koegel, R. L. (1995). Motivating communication in children with autism. In E. Schopler & G. B. Mesibov (Eds.), *Learning and cognition in autism* (pp. 73–87). Springer. https://doi.org/10.1007/978-1-4899-1286-2_5

Lamptey, R. N. L., Chaulagain, B., Trivedi, R., Gothwal, A., Layek, B., & Singh, J. A. (2022). Review of the common neurodegenerative disorders: Current therapeutic approaches and the potential role of nanotherapeutics. *International Journal of Molecular Sciences, 23*(3), 1851. https://doi.org/10.3390/ijms23031851

Lillo, P., & Hodges, J. R. (2010). Cognition and behaviour in motor neurone disease. *Current Opinion in Neurology, 23*(6), 638–642. https://doi.org/10.1097/WCO.0b013e3283400b41

Logroscino, G., Piccininni, M., Marin, B., Nichols, E., Abd-Allah, F., Abdelalim, A., Alahdab, F., Asgedom, S. W., Awasthi, A., Chaiah, Y., Daryani, A., Do, H. P., Dubey, M., Elbaz, A., Eskandarieh, S., Farhadi, F., Farzadfar, F., Fereshtehnejad, S.-M., Fernades, E., Filip, I., & Murray, C. J. L. (2018). Global, regional, and national burden of motor neuron diseases 1990-2016: A systematic analysis of the global burden of disease study 2016. *Lancet Neurology, 17*(12), 1083–1097. https://doi.org/10.1016/S1474-4422(18)30404-6

Lovaas, O. I., Koegel, R. L., & Schreibman, L. (1979). Stimulus overselectivity in autism: A review of research. *Psychological Bulletin, 86*, 1236–1254. https://doi.org/10.1037/0033-2909.86.6.1236

Luitwieler, N., Luijkx, J., Salavati, M., Van der Schans, C. P., Van der Putten, A. J., & Waninge, A. (2021). Variables related to the quality of life of families that have a child with severe to profound intellectual disabilities: A systematic review. *Heliyon, 7*, e07372. https://doi.org/10.1016/j.heliyon.2021.e07372

MacMillan, D. L., & Cauffiel, S. R. (1977). Outerdirectedness as a function of success and failure in educationally handicapped boys. *Journal of Learning Disabilities, 10*(10), 643–654. https://doi.org/10.1177/002221947701001011

Maenner, M. J., Blumberg, S. J., Kogen, M. D., Christensen, D., Yeargin-Allsopp, M., & Schieve, L. A. (2016). Prevalence of cerebral palsy and intellectual disability among children identified in two U.S. national surveys, 2011-2013. *Annals of Epidemiology, 26*, 222–226. https://doi.org/10.1016/j.annepidem.2016.01.001

Matson, J. L., Carlisle, C. B., & Bamburg, J. W. (1998). The convergent validity of the Matson evaluation of social skills for individuals with severe retardation (MESSIER). *Research in Developmental Disabilities, 19*(6), 493–500. https://doi.org/10.1016/S0891-4222(98)00020-1

Maulik, P. K., Mascarenhas, M. N., Mathers, C. D., Dua, T., & Saxena, S. (2011). Prevalence of intellectual disability: A meta-analysis of population-based studies. *Research in Developmental Disabilities, 32*(2), 419–436. https://doi.org/10.1016/j.ridd.2010.12.018

McIntyre, S., Goldsmith, S., Webb, A., Ehlinger, V., Julsen Hollung, S., McConnell, K., Arnaud, C., Smithers-Sheedy, H., Oskoui, M., Khandaker, G., Himmelmann, K., & The Global CP Prevalence Group. (2022). Global prevalence of cerebral palsy: A systematic review. *Developmental Medicine & Child Neurology, 64*(12), 1494–1506. https://doi.org/10.1111/dmcn.15346

McKinlay, A., Grace, R. C., Horwood, L. J., Fergusson, D. M., Rider, E. M., & MacFarlane, M. R. (2008). Prevalence of traumatic brain injury among children, adolescents and young adults: Prospective evidence from a birth cohort. *Brain Injury, 22*(2), 175–181. https://doi.org/10.1080/02699050801888824

Ncube, B. L., Perry, A., & Weiss, J. A. (2018). The quality of life of children with severe developmental disabilities. *Journal of Intellectual Disability Research, 62*(3), 237–244. https://doi.org/10.1111/jir.12460

Neece, C. L., Baker, B. L., Blacher, J., & Crnic, K. A. (2011). Attention-deficit/hyperactivity disorder among children with and without intellectual disability: An examination across time. *Journal of Intellectual Disability Research, 55*, 623–635. https://doi.org/10.1111/j.1365-2788.2011.01416.x

O'Reilly, G., & Carr, A. (2016). Intelligence. In A. Carr, C. Linehan, G. O'Reilly, P. Noonan Walsh, & J. McEvoy (Eds.), *The handbook of intellectual disability and clinical psychology practice* (2nd ed., pp. 81–106). Routledge.

Oskoui, M., Coutinho, F., Dykeman, J., Jetté, N., & Pringsheim, T. (2013). An update on the prevalence of cerebral palsy: A systematic review and meta-analysis. *Developmental Medicine and Child Neurology, 55*, 509–519. https://doi.org/10.1111/dmcn.12080

Plavnick, J. B. (2012). A practical strategy for teaching a child with autism to attend to and imitate a portable video model. *Research and Practice for Persons with Severe Disabilities, 37*(4), 263–270. https://doi.org/10.2511/027494813805327250

Qui, C., Kivipelto, M., & van Strauss, E. (2009). Epidemiology of Alzheimer's disease: Occurrence, determinants, and strategies toward intervention. *Dialogues in Clinical Neuroscience, 11*(2), 111–128. https://doi.org/10.31887/DCNS.2009.11.2/cqiu

Reichle, J. (1997). Communication intervention with persons who have severe disabilities. *Journal of Special Education, 31*(1), 110–134. https://doi.org/10.1177/002246699703100110

Sigafoos, J., O'Reilly, M. F., & Lancioni, G. E. (2010). Mental retardation. In J. Thomas & M. Hersen (Eds.), *Handbook of clinical psychology competencies (HCPC): Volume III: Intervention and treatment for children and adolescents* (pp. 1245–1274). Springer. https://doi.org/10.1007/978-0-387-09757-2_45

Sigafoos, J., Green, V. A., O'Reilly, M., & Lancioni, G. E. (2020). Developmental disability. In A. J. Martin, R. A. Sperling, & K. J. Newton (Eds.), *Handbook of educational psychology and students with special needs* (pp. 173–196). Routledge.

Sigafoos, J., Roche, L., & Tait, K. (2021). Challenges in providing AAC intervention to people with profound intellectual and multiple disabilities. In B. T. Ogletree (Ed.), *Augmentative and alternative communication: Challenges and solutions* (pp. 229–252). Plural Publishing.

Silver, J. M., McAllister, T. W., & Arciniegas, D. B. (Eds.). (2019). *Textbook of traumatic brain injury* (3rd ed.). American Psychiatric Publishing.

Simmons, Z. (2013). Rehabilitation of motor neuron disease. In M. P. Barnes & D. C. Good (Eds.), *Handbook of clinical neurology* (pp. 438–498). Elsevier. https://doi.org/10.1016/B978-0-444-52901-5.00041-1

Simó-Pinatella, D., Mumbardó-Adam, C., Alomar-Kurz, E., Sugai, G., & Simonsen, B. (2019). Prevalence of challenging behaviors exhibited by children with disabilities: Mapping the literature. *Journal of Behavioral. Education, 28*(3), 323–343. https://doi.org/10.1007/s10864-019-09326-9

Skandsen, T., Finnanger, T. G., Andersson, S., Lydersen, S., Brunner, J. F., & Vik, A. (2010). Cognitive impairment 3 months after moderate and severe traumatic brain injury: A prospective follow-up study. *Archives of Physical Medicine and Rehabilitation, 91*(12), 1904–1913. https://doi.org/10.1016/j.apmr.2010.08.021

Sparrow, S. S., Cicchetti, D. V., & Sauinier, C. A. (2016). *Vineland-3 adaptive behavior scales* (3rd ed.). Pearson.

Stadskleiv, K. (2020). Cognitive functioning in children with cerebral palsy. *Developmental Medicine & Child Neurology, 62*(3), 283–289. https://doi.org/10.1111/dmcn.14463

Steppe-Jones, C., Bunner, M. R., & Karnik, D. (2014). Cerebral palsy. In C. R. Reynolds, K. J. Vannest, & E. Fletcher-Janzen (Eds.), *Encyclopedia of special education* (4th ed., pp. 491–495). John Wiley & Sons.

Tassé, M. J. (2021). Adaptive behavior and functional life skills across the lifespan: Conceptual and measurement issues. In R. Lang & P. Sturmey (Eds.), *Adaptive behavior strategies for individuals with intellectual and developmental disabilities: Evidence-based practices across the lifespan* (pp. 1–20). Springer. https://doi.org/10.1007/978-3-030-66441-1_1

Tenovuo, O., Diaz-Arrastia, R., Goldstein, L. E., Sharp, D. J., van der Naalt, J., & Zasler, N. D. (2021). Assessing the severity of traumatic brain injury—Time or a change? *Journal of Clinical Medicine, 10*, 148. https://doi.org/10.3390/jcm10010148

van Bakel, E. I., Arnaud, C., Craig, S., Michelsen, S., Pildava, S., Uldall, P., & Cans, C. (2013). Monitoring the prevalence of severe intellectual disability in children across Europe: Feasibility of a common database. *Developmental Medicine & Child Neurology, 56*(4), 361–369. https://doi.org/10.1111/dmcn.12281

van Gorp, M., Hilberink, S. R., Noten, S., Benner, J. L., Stam, H. J., van der Slot, A. M. A., & Roebroeck, M. E. (2020). Epidemiology of cerebral palsy in adulthood: A systematic review and meta-analysis of the most frequently studied outcomes. *Archives of Physical Medicine and Rehabilitation, 101*(6), 1041–1052. https://doi.org/10.1016/j.apmr.2020.01.009

Vitrikas, K., Dalton, H., & Breish, D. (2020). Cerebral palsy: An overview. *American Family Physician, 101*(4), 213–220. Accessed 12 February 2024. https://www.aafp.org/pubs/afp/issues/2020/0215/p213.pdf

Voisin, T., & Vellas, B. (2009). Diagnosis and treatment of patients with severe Alzheimer's disease. *Drugs & Aging, 26*(2), 135–144. https://doi.org/10.2165/0002512-200926020-00005

Weiner, M. F., & Lipton, A. M. (Eds.). (2012). *Clinical manual of Alzheimer disease and other dementias*. American Psychiatric Publishing.

Zeidan, J., Fombonne, E., Scorah, J., Ibrahim, A., Durkin, M. S., Saxena, S., Yusuf, A., Shih, A., & Elsabbagh, M. (2022). Global prevalence of autism: A systematic review update. *Autism Research, 15*(5), 778–790. https://doi.org/10.1002/aur.2696

Chapter 2
Communication Impairment and Assessment

Communication Impairment

Communication impairment is prevalent in people with severe disabilities, and many such individuals present with severe communication impairment. The term severe communication impairment is appropriately applied when the individual lacks sufficient speech and language to meet their everyday communication needs (Sigafoos et al., 2000) or is "permanently unable to speak because of physical, developmental, or acquired disabilities, such as cerebral palsy or severe brain injury" (Hemsley et al., 2001, p. 828). People with such extremely limited spoken language ability have also been described as nonverbal or minimally verbal (Tager-Flusberg & Kasari, 2013; Zhang et al., 2015). Following a review of terminology in this area, Koegel et al. (2020) proposed that the term nonverbal should be used when, after 18 months, the person demonstrates no consistent use of any spoken words or word approximations during standardized testing. Minimally verbal, in contrast, should be used in reference to people who have "significantly fewer [words] than expected relative to age" (p. 2968), for example, less than 5 words at 18 months and fewer than 50 words at 30 months of age. One implication arising from these proposed definitional criteria is the need for standardized assessment of the person's level of communicative functioning, particularly with respect to their spoken language development.

Severe communication impairment is highly prevalent in people with severe/profound intellectual disability. Smith et al. (2020), for example, obtained data on the communication abilities of 601 adults with varying degrees of intellectual disability. They found that 76% of the adults who had severe/profound levels of intellectual disability were unable to speak or make themselves understood when speaking. In contrast, the majority of the adults who had mild and moderate intellectual disability had little or no major communication difficulties.

J. Sigafoos et al., *Communication Strategies for People with Severe Disabilities*,
Autism and Child Psychopathology Series,
https://doi.org/10.1007/978-3-031-83807-1_2

In children with autism spectrum disorder, Osterling et al. (2001) estimated that 25% are nonverbal and likely to "remain mute their entire lives" (p. 437). Rowland (2009) highlighted the fact that up to 50% of people with ASD lack sufficient speech to meet their everyday communication needs. This higher figure of 50% probably included both individuals who would be considered nonverbal and individuals who would be considered minimally verbal.

Severe communication impairment is also fairly common in people with cerebral palsy. Zhang et al. (2015), for example, obtained data on the communication abilities of 535 children with cerebral palsy from the Quebec Cerebral Palsy Registry. These data indicated that 32.3% of the children were "unable to communicate verbally" (p. 277). Further analyses of the data revealed that the inability to communicate verbally occurred mainly in children with more severe levels of physical impairment and individuals with the spastic quadriplegic and dyskinetic (i.e., involuntary muscle movement) subtypes of cerebral palsy.

More generally, severe communication impairment has long been noted as a comorbid condition among people with a range of severely disabling conditions. Bloomberg and Johnson (1990), for example, surveyed the extent of severe communication impairment in a range of service settings (e.g., early childhood programs, disability services, nursing homes, public hospitals, and mental health facilities) in Victoria, Australia. Their results suggested that 0.12% of the clients being supported in these agencies were nonspeaking or had severe communication problems. The range of conditions associated with severe communication problems in this survey included autism spectrum disorder, cerebral palsy, intellectual disability, as well as various neurological conditions, trauma, and stroke.

Complex Communication Needs

Developing viable communication strategies for nonverbal and minimally verbal individuals with severe disability is challenging. Reichle et al. (2019) considered people who were nonverbal due to severe disability to have "complex communication needs" (p. 842). The complexity is due in part to the fact that many such individuals have combinations of cognitive, sensory, physical, and learning impairments (as highlighted in Chap. 1) in addition to having limited or no speech. Because such individuals are generally unable to rely on speech as their primary mode of communication, alternative communication strategies of the type covered in Chaps. 3–10 are indicated. As part of the overall intervention process—aimed at establishing the use of one or more alternative communication strategies —it is helpful to obtain a comprehensive assessment of the person's level of communication functioning as well as their associated abilities and impairments, such as motor control, hearing, and vision.

Purposes of Communication Assessment

Data from a comprehensive communication assessment is useful for several reasons. First, objective data on the extent of the person's level of communication impairment may facilitate diagnosis and classification. Second, objective assessment data may be required to determine eligibility for speech therapy and related services.

Third, assessment of a person's language development in the expressive, receptive, and written communication domains can help identify specific areas of strength as well as areas where skills are emerging, or are absent or significantly delayed. Indeed, Brady et al. (2016) suggested that the initial aims of a communication assessment should be to "inventory and describe the individual's communication abilities..." (p. 125). Fourth, assessment information can provide objective evidence for selecting therapy goals, designing interventions to achieve those goals, and for determining response to intervention (Muller & Brady, 2016).

A more general assessment covering motor abilities, cognitive functioning, hearing, and vision can also be helpful for designing communication interventions for people with severe disabilities. Manual signing, for example, will likely be contraindicated for individuals with limited upper limb mobility. Similarly, assessment of memory and attention might inform the selection of communication strategies that involve static/permanent displays (e.g., line drawings on a communication board) versus fleeting stimuli (e.g., manual signs and gestures). Textures or tangible symbols (see Chap. 6) may be indicated for people with certain types of vision impairment. Additionally, some initial assessments of current functioning may be used periodically throughout the intervention to assess learning of targeted communication goals.

In summary, communication assessment data can be used for a variety of purposes as summarized in Table 2.1. As discussed in the next section, communication

Table 2.1 Overview of the main purposes of communication assessment for people with severe disabilities

Purpose	Example
Diagnosis/classification	Extent of spoken language development is used to differentiate between nonverbal and minimally verbal
Determine eligibility for services	Funding for high-tech communication devices (Chap. 8) may depend on the type and degree of disability and impairment
Identify strengths and needs	Limited spoken language development indicates a need for an alternative, nonspeech communication strategy
Select therapy goals	Foundational, communication skills (e.g., calling attention to self, initiating social interaction) are prioritized for intervention when underdeveloped
Design intervention	Information on physical ability and vision can assist in the selection of a suitable communication strategy
Monitor response to intervention	Assessment data on the person's progress toward the achievement of priority goals is used to determine if the intervention procedures are effective for that individual

assessment must be sufficiently broad in scope to address the varied purposes outlined in Table 2.1. Brady et al. (2016) argued that assessment of a broad range of abilities is necessary to uncover the "complex and multiple needs of individuals with severe disabilities..." (p. 125).

Scope of Communication Assessment

The American Speech-Language-Hearing Association (2004) provided extensive guidelines for undertaking a comprehensive communication assessment. The guidelines emphasized the necessity of gathering, interpreting, and applying a wide range of assessment information as part of the overall intervention process. A comprehensive communication assessment of a person with severe disability might, for example, need to consider their diagnosis, medical history, cognitive impairments and learning characteristics, hearing, and vision, as well as their spoken and nonspoken communication. In line with these guidelines, Paul and Wilson (2009) suggested that assessment should examine aspects of language development (e.g., morphology, pragmatics, semantics, syntax), early/prelinguistic behavior (e.g., pointing, gaze, joint attention, and social smiling), the frequency and amount of communication output, and the communicative functions expressed.

Information regarding communicative forms and functions that are either present, emerging, or absent is often sought from a communication assessment. In terms of forms, individuals with severe disability may use a variety of spoken and prelinguistic forms, such as word approximations, vocalizations, reaching, pointing, moving toward or away, and natural and informal gestures. Commonly assessed communicative functions include (a) recruiting attention; (b) requesting needed objects, help, or information; (c) rejecting nonpreferred stimuli; (d) commenting on aspects of the environment; (e) responding to questions; (f) following instructions; (g) establishing joint attention; and (h) initiating, maintaining, and terminating social interactions (Beuker et al., 2013; Reichle et al., 1991; Sigafoos et al., 2023). A comprehensive communication assessment should also aim to ascertain the person's understanding or comprehension words, phrases, symbols, and gestures, that is, receptive language abilities. Assessment of receptive language is important because it "forms the foundation for competent expressive language, including literacy skills" (Muller & Brady, 2016, p. 12).

Communication Assessment Strategies

A range of strategies has been used to assess the communication abilities of people with severe disabilities. This range includes both informal and formal data gathering via interview, structured and unstructured observation, and standardized rating scales (Brady et al., 2016; Chadwick et al., 2019; Reed, 2018; Sigafoos et al., 2016).

Unstructured observations, for example, might involve recording the person's communicative acts during naturalistic activities, such as during self-care routines, peer play, or mealtimes. This approach can provide useful information on the rate at which different communication forms and functions occur spontaneously, but results will depend on the number and type of communication opportunities that arise during the observation. More structured observations, in contrast, might involve creating specific numbers and types of opportunities in a systematic manner and precisely recording the person's response to each opportunity. Data from more structured observations might reveal the extent to which different communication functions (e.g., requesting, rejecting, and commenting) are evoked by specific environmental conditions. For example, does the person reliably attempt to make a request when a preferred object is offered and, if so, how does the person do this? Such information can be useful for the purpose of selecting intervention components (e.g., discriminative stimuli, prompts, and consequences).

Standardized and norm-referenced rating scales are useful for documenting the person's overall level of communication development in relation to age-graded norms. Many such rating scales can also provide information on whether specific communication skills are present, emerging, or absent from the person's repertoire. This latter type of data can assist with diagnosis and classification as well as being useful for selecting developmentally appropriate intervention targets.

In a survey of 55 UK-based speech-language therapists, Chadwick et al. (2019) found that structured and unstructured observation were the most commonly used approaches for assessing the communication skills of the children and adults with profound intellectual and multiple disabilities that they were supporting. Specifically, 63.3% of the respondents reported conducting observation-based assessments, such as observing the child's use of everyday objects. The respondents also reported using 26 different types of published/research-based assessment instruments. The most commonly used instruments were the (a) PreVerbal Communication Schedule (Kiernan & Reid, 1987), (b) Affective Communication Assessment (Coupe et al., 1985), and (c) Triple C: Checklist of Communicative Competence (Iacono et al., 2005). These three tools (summarized in Table 2.2) were reportedly used by 45.5, 38.2, and 16.4% of the respondents, respectively. A general concern noted by the authors was the limited use of empirical evidence to "support assessment selection decisions" (p. 346). However, this concern might not be generalizable to other locales or to other respondents working with other types of clients.

In addition to the instruments listed in Table 2.2, there are numerous other standardized rating scales that have established reliability and validity for assessing minimally verbal and nonverbal people with severe disabilities. Commonly used scales in this category include the third edition of the *Vineland Adaptive Behavior Scales*™ (*Vineland-3*; Sparrow et al., 2016), the fourth edition of the Receptive-Expressive Emergent Language Scale (*REEL-4*; Bzoch & League, 2020), and the Rossetti Infant-Toddler Language Scale (Rossetti, 2005). Table 2.3 provides a summary of these three instruments.

Table 2.2 Summary of items and areas assessed by the PreVerbal Communication Schedule, Affective Communication Assessment, and the Triple C: Checklist of Communicative Competence

Instrument	Areas assessed
PreVerbal Communication Schedule (Kiernan & Reid, 1987)	Consists of 195 items covering pre-communicative behavior, imitation skills, informal communication behavior, and formal communicative behavior. Examples of skills assessed include (a) shows interest in pictures and photos, (b) recognizes visual cues, (c) imitates speech sounds, (d) points to indicate preferences, and (d) responds to own name when called. Items are rated as usually, rarely, or never occurring. Appropriate for assessing early communication development in nonverbal and minimally verbal individuals
Affective Communication Assessment (Coupe et al., 1985)	Assesses how the person indicates likes and dislikes by recording reactions to the presentation of various stimuli, such as tastes, sounds, aromas, and textures. Behavioral indicators of likes/wants and disliked/rejected stimuli could consist of various pre-intentional responses, such as a change in breathing patterns or posture, eye movements, facial expressions, vocalizations, and body movement (e.g., turning away from a tactile stimulus). This assessment is intended for use with nonverbal individuals at the pre-intentional stage of communication development
Triple C: Checklist of Communicative Competence (Iacono et al., 2005)	Consists of 20 checklists covering the presence or absence of functional and observable communication skills representing five stages of communication development: (a) pre-intentional passive communication, (b) pre-intentional active communication, (c) intentional informal communication, (d) basic symbolic communication, and (e) established symbolic communication. Intended for use in assessing nonverbal and minimally verbal adolescents and adults with severe and multiple disabilities

Table 2.3 Summary of the Vineland-3, REEL-4, and Rosetti Infant-Toddler Language Scale

Instrument	Areas assessed
Vineland-3 (Sparrow et al., 2016)	The Vineland-3 is a comprehensive norm-referenced assessment of adaptive behavior functioning across five areas: Communication, daily living, socialization, motor skills, and maladaptive behavior. The scale was normed on large, representative US samples covering birth to 90 years of age. The communication area includes assessment of 39 receptive skills, 49 expressive skills, and 38 written communication skills. Items are scored as usually, sometimes, or never performed when needed or appropriate. Results can be used to estimate the degree of delay/impairment and identify specific target skills for intervention
REEL-4 (Bzoch & League, 2020)	The REEL-4 is a standardized norm-referenced rating scale based on 1019 infants and toddlers matched to the 2019 US population. The scale consists of 76 items covering receptive and expressive language development from birth to three years of age. Items are scored as typical of the child's behavior (+), not observed (−), or partly observed/emerging (±). Scores can distinguish typically developing children from children with receptive and expressive impairments associated with autism and developmental delay/disability

(continued)

Table 2.3 (continued)

Instrument	Areas assessed
Rosetti Infant-Toddler Language Scale (Rossetti, 2005)	This is a criterion-referenced instrument that assesses skills related to six areas of communicative functioning: Interaction-attachment, pragmatics, use of gestures, play behavior, comprehension, and expressive communication. Items are arranged into age groups from birth to 3 years. Items are scored as either observed spontaneously, directly elicited, or as not observed/elicited. Administration can occur via direct (unstructured or structured) observation or by interviewing parents/caregivers. The main purpose of the scale is to identify problems with respect to the child's pre-verbal and verbal-language development

Behavior-Analytic Assessment Instruments

Sigafoos et al. (2023) reviewed communication assessments derived from a behavior-analytic orientation and based on Skinner's (1957) functional analysis of communication behavior. A unique aspect of the behaviorally oriented instruments reviewed by Sigafoos et al. (2023) is that these instruments tend to consider both spoken and nonspoken communicative forms or behaviors, as well as a range of functional communication skills, such as requesting, rejecting, commenting, responding to questions, and imitation of communication behavior. This type of information is highly relevant because these types of functional communication skills (both spoken and nonspoken forms of communication) are considered developmentally appropriate and of direct benefit to the individual. The potential direct benefits of targeting functional communication skills include the fact that such skills will likely enable the person to express important wants and needs and more generally exert a degree of control over the environment (Reichle et al., 1991).

Instruments in this category that have been empirically validated for assessing the functional communication abilities of nonverbal and minimally verbal people with severe disabilities include (a) the Behavioral Language Assessment Form (Sundberg & Partington, 1998), (b) the Verbal Behavior Assessment Scale (Duker, 1999), and (c) the Verbal Behavior Milestones Assessment and Placement Program (Sundberg, 2014). Table 2.4 summarizes the key features of these three instruments.

Summary and Conclusion

Severe communication impairment is prevalent among people with severe disabilities, and many individuals with severe disabilities meet the definition of nonverbal or minimally verbal. These individuals generally cannot rely on spoken language to meet their everyday communication needs and should therefore receive intervention aimed at teaching them to use one or more of the alternative communication strategies covered in Chapters 3–10. This does not mean that efforts to establish speech should not be made. Rather, it suggests that practitioners should also aim to establish functional use of alternative (i.e., nonspeech) communication modes.

Table 2.4 Key features of the Behavioral Language Assessment Form, Verbal Behavior Assessment Scale, and Verbal Behavior Milestones Assessment and Placement Program

Instrument	Key features
Behavioral Language Assessment Form (BLAF; Sundberg & Partington, 1998)	This 60-question scale assesses requesting and rejecting functions as well as vocal imitation, naming, topical conversational skills, cooperation, motor imitation, and matching abilities. Results provide a profile of communication forms and functions. Results are used to inform intervention design and sequencing
Verbal Behavior Assessment Scale (Duker, 1999)	This 15-question scale assesses the strength of three basic communicative functions: Requesting, naming, and imitation. Both spoken and nonverbal modes (e.g., use of gestures) are assessed. Results are used to identify functional deficits and select target skills
Verbal Behavior Milestones Assessment and Placement Program (Sundberg, 2014)	Focuses on early (birth to 4 years) communication development and four basic communicative functions (i.e., requesting/rejecting, naming/commenting, imitative communication, and conversation/thematic responding). Social play and basic academic skills are also assessed. Results can be used to create profiles of strengths and deficits, select target behavior, and inform intervention

Assessing the person's communication abilities is a critical component of the overall intervention process. Assessment data are used for several purposes, including identifying existing communicative forms and functions, selecting target skills, setting intervention goals, designing intervention procedures, and evaluating intervention progress/outcomes. Assessment data can be gathered using various strategies and instruments, including structured and unstructured observations and formal/standardized rating scales. A comprehensive assessment covering expressive and receptive speech and language development and the communicative forms and functions present or absent from the person's repertoire will typically require a highly individualized and flexible approach that makes use of a combination of strategies.

References

American Speech-Language-Hearing Association. (2004). *Preferred practice patterns for the profession of speech-language pathology [Preferred Practice Patterns]*. Retrieved from www.asha.org/policy/. https://doi.org/10.1044/policy.PP2004-00191 on 20 March 2024.

Beuker, K. T., Rommelse, N. N. J., Danders, R., & Buitelaar, J. K. (2013). Development of early communication skills in the first two years of life. *Infant Behavior and Development, 36*(1), 71–83. https://doi.org/10.1016/j.infbeh.2012.11.001

Bloomberg, K., & Johnson, H. (1990). A statewide demographic survey of people with severe communication impairments. *Augmentative and Alternative Communication, 6*(1), 50–60. https://doi.org/10.1080/07434619012331275314

Brady, N., Bruce, S., Goldman, A., Erickson, K., Mineo, B., Ogletree, B. T., Paul, D., Romski, M. A., Sevcik, R., Siegel, E., Schoonover, J., Snell, M., Sylvester, L., & Wilkinson, K. (2016). Communication services and supports for individuals with severe disabilities: Guidance for assessment and intervention. *American Journal of Intellectual and Developmental Disabilities, 121*(2), 121–138. https://doi.org/10.1352/1944-7558-121.2.121

Bzoch, K., & League, R. (2020). *Receptive expressive emergent language scales—Revised (REEL-4)* (4th ed.). Pro-Ed.

Chadwick, D., Buell, S., & Goldbart, J. (2019). Approaches to communication assessment with children and adults with profound intellectual and multiple disabilities. *Journal of Applied Research in Intellectual Disabilities, 32*(2), 336–358. https://doi.org/10.1111/jar.12530

Coupe, J., Barton, L., Collins, L., Levy, D., & Murphy, D. (1985). *The affective communication assessment*. Manchester Education. Retrieved 25 March 2024 from: http://complexneeds.org.uk/modules/Module-2.4-Assessment-monitoring-and-evaluation/All/m08p020b.html

Duker, P. C. (1999). The verbal behavior assessment scale (VerBAS): Construct validity, reliability, and internal consistency. *Research in Developmental Disabilities, 20*(5), 347–353. https://doi.org/10.1016/s0891-4222(99)00016-5

Hemsley, B., Sigafoos, J., Balandin, S., Forbes, R., Taylor, C., Green, V. A., & Parmenter, T. (2001). Nursing the patient with severe communication impairment. *Journal of Advanced Nursing, 35*(6), 827–835. https://doi.org/10.1046/j.1365-2648.2001.01920.x

Iacono, T., Bloomberg, K., & West, D. (2005). A preliminary investigation into the internal consistency and construct validity of the triple C: Checklist of communicative competencies. *Journal of Intellectual and Developmental Disabilities, 30*(3), 127–138. https://doi.org/10.1080/13668250500204059

Kiernan, C., & Reid, B. (1987). *Preverbal communication schedule (PVCS)*. Retrieved on 25 March 2024 from: http://complexneeds.org.uk/modules/Module-2.4-Assessment-monitoring-and-evaluation/B/downloads/m08p030b/the_pvcs.pdf

Koegel, L. K., Bryan, K. M., Su, P. L., Vaidya, M., & Camarata, S. (2020). Definitions of nonverbal and minimally verbal in research for autism: A systematic review of the literature. *Journal of Autism and Developmental Disorders, 50*(8), 2957–2972. https://doi.org/10.1007/s10803-020-04402-w

Muller, K., & Brady, N. (2016). Assessing early receptive language skills in children with ASD. *Perspectives of the ASHA Special Interest Groups, 1*(1), 12–19. https://doi.org/10.1044/persp1.SIG1.12

Osterling, J., Dawson, G., & McPartland, J. (2001). Autism. In C. E. Walker & M. C. Roberts (Eds.), *Handbook of clinical child psychology* (3rd ed., pp. 432–452). John Wiley & Sons.

Paul, R., & Wilson, K. P. (2009). Assessing speech, language, and communication in autism spectrum disorders. In S. Goldstein, J. A. Naglieri, & S. Ozanoff (Eds.), *Assessment of autism spectrum disorders* (5th ed., pp. 171–208). Guilford Press.

Reed, V. A. (2018). *An introduction to children with language disorders* (5th ed.). Pearson.

Reichle, J., York, J., & Sigafoos, J. (1991). *Implementing augmentative and alternative communication: Strategies for learners with severe disabilities*. Paul H. Brookes Publishing Co.

Reichle, J., Simacek, J., Wattanawongwan, S., & Ganz, J. (2019). Implementing aided augmentative communication systems with persons having complex communication needs. *Behavior Modification, 43*(6), 841–878. https://doi.org/10.1177/0145445519858272

Rossetti, L. (2005). *Rossetti Infant-Toddler Language Scale*. LinguiSystems.

Rowland, C. M. (2009). Presymbolic communicators with autism spectrum disorders. In P. Mirenda & T. Iacono (Eds.), *Autism spectrum disorders and AAC* (pp. 51–81). Paul H. Brookes Publishing Co.

Sigafoos, J., Woodyatt, G., Keen, D., Tait, K., Tucker, M., Roberts-Pennell, D., & Pittendreigh, N. (2000). Identifying potential communicative acts in children with developmental and physical disabilities. *Communication Disorders Quarterly, 21*(2), 77–86. https://doi.org/10.1177/152574010002100202

Sigafoos, J., Lancioni, G. E., O'Reilly, M. F., Lang, R., Singh, N. N., Didden, R., Green, V. A., & Marschik, P. B. (2016). Communication. In N. N. Singh (Ed.), *Handbook of evidence-based practices in intellectual and developmental disabilities* (pp. 823–850). Springer. https://doi.org/10.1007/978-3-319-26583-4_31

Sigafoos, J., Carnett, A., Schlosser, R. W., O'Reilly, M. F., & Lancioni, G. E. (2023). Communication assessment and intervention. In J. L. Matson (Ed.), *Handbook of applied behavior analysis for children with autism* (pp. 109–127). Springer. https://doi.org/10.1007/978-3-031-27587-6_9
Skinner, B. F. (1957). *Verbal behavior*. Prentice-Hall.
Smith, M., Manduchi, B., Burke, E., Carroll, R., McCallion, P., & McCarron, M. (2020). Communication difficulties in adults with intellectual disabilities. *Research in Developmental Disabilities, 97*(103557). https://doi.org/10.1016/j.ridd.2019.103557
Sparrow, S. S., Cicchetti, D. V., & Saulnier, C. A. (2016). *Vineland adaptive behavior scales™ (Vineland-3)* (3rd ed.). Pearson.
Sundberg, M. L. (2014). *VB-MAPP: Verbal behavior milestones assessment and placement program: A language and social skills assessment program for children with autism or other developmental disabilities*. AVB Press.
Sundberg, M. L., & Partington, J. W. (1998). *Teaching language to children with autism or other developmental disabilities*. Behavior Analysts, Inc.
Tager-Flusberg, H., & Kasari, C. (2013). Minimally verbal school-aged children with autism spectrum disorder: The neglected end of the spectrum. *Autism Research, 6*(6), 468–478. https://doi.org/10.1002/aur.1329
Zhang, J. Y., Oskoui, M., & Shevell, M. (2015). A population-based study of communication impairment in cerebral palsy. *Journal of Child Neurology, 30*(3), 277–284. https://doi.org/10.1177/0883073814538497

Chapter 3
Prelinguistic Communication

Introduction

In the language acquisition literature, a distinction is commonly made between prelinguistic and linguistic stages of communication development (Wetherby et al., 1998). The prelinguistic stage covers the period from birth to about 10–12 months of age (Zhang et al., 2024). This early period is characterized by the gradual emergence and development of various prelinguistic behaviors (e.g., crying, cooing, gaze, facial expressions, gestures, and body language) into more readily recognized and intentional communicative acts (Iverson & Wozniak, 2016). Additional abilities that typically emerge during the prelinguistic stage of communication development—that might facilitate transition to the linguistic stage of development—include joint attending, social turn-taking, interactive play skills, verbal reciprocity, and imitation (Toth et al., 2006). The development of prelinguistic behaviors into intentional forms of communication has been attributed, in part, to the fact that parents frequently respond contingently to the presumed meaning, intent, purpose, or function of their child's prelinguistic acts (Jeon & Lee, 2023; Lopez et al., 2020).

From 10 months of age onward, the quantity and complexity of the typically developing child's language, both expressive and receptive, increase. For example, the first few recognizable words appear at around 10–12 months of age (Frank et al., 2017). From then on, spoken language increasingly comes to replace the child's prior reliance on prelinguistic behavior. This typical course of development is rarely seen in children who present with severe disability from an early age.

Nonverbal and minimally verbal children with severe disability often continue to function at a prelinguistic or even pre-intentional stage well past the age when other children are rapidly developing spoken language (Crais & Ogletree, 2016). In fact, some children with severe disability may never develop any appreciable amount of speech as noted in Chap. 2. Some such individuals may thus come to rely almost exclusively on prelinguistic forms of behavior to communicate.

J. Sigafoos et al., *Communication Strategies for People with Severe Disabilities*, Autism and Child Psychopathology Series,
https://doi.org/10.1007/978-3-031-83807-1_3

Sigafoos et al. (2000), for example, collected data on the communication forms and functions used by 20 children and adolescents with developmental disability and severe communication impairment. All 20 children (aged 16 months to 15 years of age) were reported by parents and teachers to communicate primarily via prelinguistic behaviors, such as through vocalizations, body movements, facial expressions, and by looking at wanted or needed objects. In some cases, children were reported to communicate through problematic forms of behavior, such as tantrums, aggression, and self-injurious behavior. Use of linguistic forms (e.g., spoken words or manual signing) was rarely reported. The prelinguistic acts reportedly used by these children were often interpreted by parents and teachers as the child's means of communicating a number of different functions, purposes, or intents, including being used to greet others, request objects, indicate dislikes, recruit attention, and comment. The study revealed that parents and teachers often viewed their child's prelinguistic behaviors as if these were indeed intentional communicative acts. However, Sigafoos et al. (2006) cautioned that prelinguistic behaviors may or may not represent intentional forms of communication. Given this uncertainty, prelinguistic behaviors present in the child's repertoire might be more cautiously viewed as having communicative potential. That potential might be realized through intervention aimed at enabling the person to communicate specific functions (e.g., requesting, joint attention, rejecting/protesting) more clearly using socially appropriate prelinguistic behaviors.

Numerous investigators have documented the predominance of prelinguistic communication acts (e.g., using vocalizations, gestures, and/or facial expressions to request, protest, and/or comment) in the repertoires of children with severe disabilities (Iacono et al., 1998; Liu et al., 2024; McLean & Synder-McLean, 1987). Didden et al. (2010), for example, surveyed the communication forms and functions reportedly used by 120 children and adults with Rett syndrome. Rett syndrome is a genetic disorder affecting predominately females and resulting in severe/profound levels of cognitive and physical impairment, including severe communication impairment in most cases. As in the Sigafoos et al. (2000) study, most of the 120 participants in Didden et al.'s survey reportedly relied primarily on prelinguistic forms (mainly eye gaze) to achieve a few basic communication functions. The foremost communication functions referenced included choice making, recruiting attention, and responding to others. Didden et al. also found that 10–41% of these participants reportedly engaged in problematic behavior (e.g., yelling/screaming and self-injury) that were interpreted as intentional communicative acts. Several lines of evidence show that problematic forms of prelinguistic behavior can serve a range of communicative functions (e.g., recruit attention, request preferred objects, and reject nonpreferred stimuli) for people with severe disabilities who are nonverbal or minimally verbal (Reichle & Wacker, 2017; Sigafoos et al., 2016).

Given that many children with severe disability appear to function at the prelinguistic stage, efforts to enhance their prelinguistic skills could be seen as a logical intervention approach. For some individuals, prelinguistic behavior may represent a viable and effective communication strategy. Intervention focused on strengthening the person's prelinguistic skills might, for example, enable the person to achieve meaningful outcomes (e.g., social interaction, access to preferred or needed objects, and self-determined choices).

Use of prelinguistic communication strategies could be seen as a reasonable alternative when the probability of speech and language developing is minimal or as an initial form of intervention to enhance speech and language development. Intervention focused on boosting the clarity and consistency of the child's prelinguistic signaling would also be relevant in cases where the meaning of the child's existing communicative attempts via prelinguistic behaviors is difficult for listeners to detect and interpret. As noted by Keen (2014), reliance on prelinguistic forms may be limiting if the forms used are difficult for listeners to detect and interpret. For other individuals, establishment of effective prelinguistic skills might facilitate the transition to more developmentally advanced linguistic/symbolic forms of communication. Crais and Ogletree (2016), for example, suggested that communication-related gains at the prelinguistic stage could be foundational for later development of spoken language and sign-based communication.

Review of Prelinguistic Intervention Research

Numerous studies have evaluated the effects of various types of prelinguistic interventions on the communication functioning of people with severe disabilities. The accumulated research has been synthesized in three recent high-quality systematic reviews (Dubin & Lieberman-Betz, 2020; McDaniel et al., 2022; Peters-Scheffer et al., 2016). All three reviews focused on evaluating intervention studies aimed at enhancing the prelinguistic skills of children with autism or developmental delay/disability. Table 3.1 summarizes each of these three reviews in terms of number of studies included, participants, types of prelinguistic interventions that were evaluated, and the main findings/conclusions arising from the synthesis of the included studies.

Peters-Scheffer et al. (2016)

In their 2016 review, Peters-Scheffer et al. identified 23 studies that evaluated the effects of one specific type of prelinguistic intervention, that is, Prelinguistic Milieu Teaching (PMT). PMT focuses on increasing functional use of prelinguistic communication forms (e.g., vocalizations and gestures). PMT also often targets joint attending skills. Joint attention refers to the act of shifting one's gaze between some object or aspect of the environment and a communicative partner in a bid to access the object and/or direct the communicative partner's attention toward the stimulus of interest. PMT is premised on the hypothesis that increasing the frequency and clarity of meaning of the child's prelinguistic skills, including joint attending skills,

Table 3.1 Summary of three recent systematic reviews of prelinguistic intervention studies

Review citation	Number of studies	Participants	Interventions	Findings/conclusion
Peters-Scheffer et al. (2016)	23	315 children (1–8 years of age) with developmental delay/disorders	Prelinguistic milieu teaching	Prelinguistic milieu Teaching increases prelinguistic communication in children with developmental disorders
Dubin and Lieberman-Betz (2020)	25	387 children (1–8 years) with autism spectrum disorder	10 different types of naturalistic procedures/ programs	Naturalistic intervention increases prelinguistic behavior and promotes generalization and maintenance
McDaniel et al. (2022)	68	1040 children (mean age 3.5–4.5 years) with autism spectrum disorder	36+ different types of responsivity intervention strategies	Responsivity intervention strategies can improve the prelinguistic skills and language abilities of children with autism spectrum disorder

may not only increase the child's communicative success, but might also facilitate the emergence of more advanced linguistic/symbolic forms of communication.

In terms of implementation, PMT is typically delivered in naturalistic and one-on-one play-based sessions. The key procedural components of PMT include (a) arranging the environment to create the need for the child to initiate a communicative act, (b) following the child's lead, and (c) establishing social, turn-taking/play routines. For example, a child's favorite toy might be placed in sight, but out to reach to create the need for the child to initiate a [prelinguistic] request. A child's prelinguistic request might consist of reaching for the toy while also vocalizing or perhaps shifting their gaze from the toy to the communication partner and back again. In response to such initiations, the communicative partner reinforces the act by giving the child the toy. The partner then further engages with the play routine, such as by imitating the child's play actions, while also making relevant comments. As the play session proceeds, the partner creates additional teaching opportunities by momentarily interrupting or changing the social-play routine to evoke additional and novel initiations of requests or comments from the child. The general PMT approach could be seen as a variation and refinement of more general incidental teaching procedures that have been successfully used to increase the frequency and complexity of speech in children with language delay (Hart & Risley, 1975).

The 23 PMT studies identified by Peters-Scheffer et al. (2016) provided intervention to a total of 315 children. Most of the participating children, who ranged from 1:5 to 8:0 (years:months), were classified as having a developmental delay, but studies also included children with more specific diagnoses, such as cerebral palsy, prematurity, failure to thrive, autism spectrum disorder, and other syndromes (e.g., Angelman, Downs, Fragile X, and fetal alcohol syndrome). Most of these 315 participants would likely be classified as prelinguistic communicators because they were functioning at the 9–15-month level in terms of overall communication development.

In terms of intervention delivery, the modal pattern in the 23 studies reviewed by Peters-Scheffer et al. (2016) was for the researchers to schedule from 3 to 4 sessions per week, with each session lasting from 20 to 60 min. However, a few studies were designed to compare the effects of providing differing amounts of intervention (e.g., 1 versus 5 hrs per week). The time span over which intervention was provided ranged from 7 weeks to 9 months. Thus, in a program consisting of 2 hrs per week for 7 weeks, children would receive 14 total intervention hours, whereas in a 9-month program, some 72 intervention hours would be delivered.

In terms of the outcomes from the 23 studies reviewed by Peters-Scheffer et al. (2016), the overall findings indicated that PMT intervention was associated with improvement in the participating children's prelinguistic communication behavior as evidenced by, for example, (a) increased initiation of requests and comments, (b) increases in the overall frequency of communication, and (c) improvement with respect to the clarity of the child's communicative signals and the extent to which the meaning of the child's communicative attempts was successfully conveyed to their communicative partners. Some studies also reported that children developed more advanced, linguistic/symbolic forms to initiate communication. Additional positive outcomes reported in some studies included increased social interaction and improved play skills.

Based on their analysis of these 23 studies, Peters-Scheffer et al. (2016) concluded that "PMT is a promising approach for increasing the communication of children with developmental disabilities" (p. 170). However, the authors further noted that the extent to which positive outcomes accrue may depend on the responsivity of the parents/play partners. A variation of PMT exists in which partners are also trained to identify the child's often subtle communicative attempts and to be more responsive to these attempts. This variation (known as Responsivity Education/Prelinguistic Milieu Teaching or RE/PMT) is indicated when parents are relatively less responsive initially to their child's prelinguistic communicative attempts (Fey et al., 2006). Overall, the Peters-Scheffer et al. review indicates that there is sufficient empirical evidence to support the use of PMT for increasing the prelinguistic skills of young children with developmental delay/disabilities.

To supplement the Peters-Scheffer et al. (2016) review, an interesting case study by McCathren (2000) is described in Box 3.1. This case study is presented to illustrate the implementation and evaluation of a PMT intervention for an individual child. A unique aspect of the McCathren study is the fact that the PMT intervention was successfully delivered by the child's teacher in the classroom. This is significant because the study provides some evidence that PMT can be successfully implemented under real-world conditions.

Box 3.1 Summary of McCathren's (2000) PMT Intervention Study

McCathren (2000) evaluated the effects of a PMT intervention provided to a 3.5-year-old boy. The boy (Michael) was described as nonverbal and as having limited imitation ability and communicative intentionality. Michael had not responded to previous efforts aimed at teaching him to use sign language. The aim of intervention was to increase intentional communication. Intentional communication was defined as use of a conventional word, sign, or gesture (e.g., waving, head nod, pointing). Intentional communication included establishing joint attention using an adult-to-object-to-adult gaze shift. Intervention was primarily directed at two communicative functions, that is, behavior regulation (i.e., requesting) and directing the adult's attention to an environmental stimulus. Following initial baseline phases, the teacher provided PMT intervention aimed first at increasing intentional communication and eye contact. In later intervention phases, vocalizations and symbolic/conventional gestures were targeted for increase. For intervention, the teacher was trained to implement six general tactics associated with PMT and related naturalistic/incidental teaching procedures: (a) following the child's lead, (b) response prompting (e.g., prompting eye contact by instructing the child to *Look at me*.), (c) imitating the child's physical actions and vocalizations, (d) modeling communication, such as by pointing to out-of-reach objects, (e) engaging the child in turn-taking play routines, and (f) environmental arrangement (e.g., placing highly preferred objects in sight but out of reach to induce a request). Data on the dependent variables were collected during two, 20-min weekly sessions. Over the course of intervention, Michael showed a noticeable increase in the frequency of intentional communicative acts, including increased eye contact and vocalizations. There was also some increase in the use of more advanced/symbolic communication forms (i.e., vocalizations with consonants and conventional gestures). The results suggest that the teacher's implementation of the PMT intervention was effective in increasing Michael's initiation of intentional communication using prelinguistic behaviors. The intervention also increased the use of more advanced/conventional communication responses. The positive intervention effects reported by McCathren (2000) are consistent with the general findings from the Peters-Scheffer et al. (2016) review of PMT studies.

Dubin and Lieberman-Betz

The Dubin and Lieberman-Betz (2020) review could be seen as more inclusive than the review conducted by Peters-Scheffer et al. (2016) because it sought out studies evaluating a wider range of prelinguistic interventions, not just PMT. Specifically,

Dubin and Lieberman-Betz selected for review studies that used any type of child-focused/naturalistic approach to improve aspects of prelinguistic communication. On the other hand, they limited their search to studies targeting prelinguistic behaviors (e.g., gestures, gaze shifts, and vocalizations) related to three main communicative functions: (a) initiating joint attention, (c) initiating a request, and (c) initiating social interaction. The search was also limited to studies involving young children with autism spectrum disorder.

Dubin and Lieberman-Betz's (2020) search yielded 25 studies. These 25 studies provided intervention to a total of 387 children (1–8 years of age). Eight main types of child-focused/naturalistic interventions were represented across these 25 studies. Table 3.2 lists and briefly describes the features of the eight main types of intervention programs represented in Dubin and Lieberman-Betz's review. In addition to the formally named approaches described in Table 3.2, the independent variable in

Table 3.2 Interventions represented in the Dubin and Lieberman-Betz (2020) review

Intervention	Description
ASAP[a]	Manualized program for autistic preschoolers. Targets social interaction, requesting, and joint attention. Involves following the child's lead, natural reinforcement, incidental teaching, and response prompting (Dykstra et al., 2012)
ESI[a]	Parent-implemented program for autistic toddlers. Targets social communication. Naturalistic strategies are embedded into everyday routines (Wetherby & Woods, 2006)
IS[a]	Targets social imitation, joint attention, and shared positive affect. Emphasizes "opportunities to respond to and initiate joint attention, imitate others during social interaction, and share positive affect, with interventionists enticing and modeling social targets, prompting as needed" (Landa et al., 2011, p. 4)
JASPER[a]	Play-based intervention to improve social communication. Targets joint attention, engagement, and behavioral regulation. Involves natural contexts, following the child's lead, natural reinforcement, modeling, and prompting (Kasari et al., 2021)
PMT[a]	Naturalistic intervention focusing on increasing prelinguistic vocalizations, gestures, and joint attention bids. Procedures embedded in social/turn-taking/play routines include environmental arrangement and following the child's lead (Peters-Scheffer et al., 2016)
PRT[a]	Targets motivation, responding to multiple cues, self-management, and self-initiation. Involves following the child's lead, offering choice, prompting attending, structured opportunities within turn-taking routines, interspersed maintenance and acquisition trials, response shaping, and natural reinforcement (Koegel & Koegel, 2006)
CI[a]	Embeds high-interest materials to increase initiation of joint attention bids. Prompting, prompt fading, and reinforcement are also used (Kryzak & Jones, 2015)
RIT[a]	Naturalistic developmental behavior intervention that targets imitation during play. Therapist uses simplified language, gestures, modeling, imitation, and expansion (Ingersoll, 2010)

[a]*Note*: *ASAP* Advancing Social-Communication and Play, *ESI* Early Social Interaction Project, *IS* Interpersonal synchrony, *JASPER* Joint Attention and Symbolic Play Engagement and Regulation, *PMT* Prelinguistic Milieu Teaching, *PRT* Pivotal Response Training, *CI* circumscribed interests, *RIT* Reciprocal Imitation Training

these 25 studies generally also included the application of a range of well-established intervention procedures, such as response prompting, prompt fading, natural reinforcement, modeling, imitation, and expansion.

Most studies reviewed by Dubin and Lieberman-Betz (2020) aimed to increase children's use of gaze shift, gestures, and/or vocalizations to establish joint attention and make requests. In all 25 studies, intervention involved a one-to-one delivery mode, although three studies also ran some group-based sessions. In about half the studies, the intervention agents were the child's parents and/or regular teaching personnel, but other studies had therapists or university/research personnel implementing the procedures. Intervention duration ranged from 5 to 52 weeks, but most studies provided intervention over a period of about 8–12 weeks.

The unifying characteristic of the studies in the Dubin and Lieberman-Betz (2020) review was that they all generally adhered to the naturalistic developmental behavioral paradigm outlined by Schreibman et al. (2015). Naturalistic developmental behavioral approaches are characterized by four major intervention components: (a) embedding teaching opportunities into natural routines, (b) following the child's lead, (c) use of natural reinforcement, and (d) use of various behavioral teaching procedures, such as response prompting, prompt fading, time delay, behavior chain interruption, and response shaping. Prelinguistic interventions also often supplement these four main components with additional instructional tactics, such as arranging the environment to tempt or induce communication, modeling desired communicative acts, imitating the child's actions, verbal narration of the child's behavior, and expanding child initiations.

Based on their synthesis of the results from these 25 studies, Dubin and Lieberman-Betz (2020) concluded that the literature overall offers promising evidence for the efficacy of naturalistic prelinguistic interventions. Dubin and Lieberman-Betz's analyses showed that these interventions were generally effective for increasing prelinguistic behaviors (e.g., gesture, vocalization, and gaze shift) related to the communicative functions of joint attention, requesting, and initiating social interaction.

A factor that does somewhat limit the results of the Dubin and Lieberman-Betz's (2020) review is the relative absence of comparison studies that would enable clinicians to determine which specific brand of prelinguistic intervention described in Table 3.2 might be best suited to any given individual or setting. In some respects, decisions related to which specific prelinguistic intervention to use might not be all that critical given that these types of interventions share many components and generally adhere to the same set of underlying instructional principles, as described by Schreibman et al. (2015). It is possible, therefore, that the efficacy of prelinguistic intervention may depend more on how well the core set of underlying instructional principles are implemented rather than on any idiosyncratic feature of a particular program.

McDaniel et al. (2022)

The final review summarized in Table 3.1 was the most comprehensive in that it covered 68 studies that collectively involved 1040 children and 36 different intervention programs. McDaniel et al. (2022) focused on studies evaluating what they referred to as "responsivity intervention strategies." Responsivity intervention strategies were defined as "strategies designed to support the development of turn-taking conversations through setting up the environment to increase communication by following the child's lead, using natural reinforcement for communicative attempts, and providing targeted input" (p. 4784). This definition indicates that responsivity intervention strategies incorporate the same general instructional strategies found in other prelinguistic interventions (e.g., environmental arrangement, following the child's lead, natural reinforcement, and response prompting). McDaniel et al. acknowledged the close relation between responsivity intervention strategies and the more general naturalistic developmental and behavioral approach to intervention.

Within the 68 studies reviewed by McDaniel et al. (2022), the most frequently cited interventions used were JASPER and PRT (see Table 3.2), but collectively these two programs were only used in a total of 14 studies. This means that the large number of remaining studies employed some other form of responsivity intervention. This variety would seem to complicate any attempt to tease out the relative effects of the many different and specific types of programs. However, as noted above, the specific program used might be of little relevance given that these interventions are all pretty much based on the same underlying set of instructional principles as described by Schreibman et al. (2015).

As might be expected from such a comprehensive survey of the literature, a variety of dependent variables were targeted in the 68 studies reviewed by McDaniel et al. (2022). The range of outcomes measured included the fairly standard set of prelinguistic behavior reported elsewhere (e.g., joint attending, gestures/pointing, vocalizations, and imitation), but also some rather novel kinds of responses, such as conversational phrases per minute, semiotic behavior, symbolic turn-taking, and verbal reciprocity. An example of a positive outcome related to semiotic behavior is when the child learns to signal more clearly to convey or clarify the intended meaning of their communicative initiation. An example of verbal reciprocity is when there is a back-and-forth vocal exchange between parent and child and when the child's response to the parent's speech might involve a contingent vocalization. The interesting mix of dependent variables might indicate that researchers are expanding the range of skills or abilities that are considered important for intervention.

The amount and duration of intervention varied as did the manner in which researchers reported these aspects of their method. Generally, studies reported the amount and duration of intervention in terms of minutes of intervention per session, sessions per week, and/or total number of intervention weeks. A typical delivery approach involved anywhere from 12 to 30 intervention sessions with each session lasting about 20–30 min, and with sessions spread out over 6–12 weeks. A rough estimate is that a child would typically receive about 20–30 h of intervention when participating in one of these responsivity intervention studies.

Overall, the literature reviewed by McDaniel et al. (2022) provides good empirical evidence to support the use of responsivity intervention strategies for enhancing prelinguistic skills and several language-related skills in young children with autism spectrum disorder. In this respect, the results are consistent with the conclusions reached by Dubin and Lieberman-Betz (2020) and Peters-Scheffer et al. (2016). The consistency of outcomes across the three major reviews considered in this chapter is perhaps not surprising given that, as noted previously, these types of prelinguistic interventions have all incorporated the same general components associated with the naturalistic developmental behavioral intervention approach outlined by Schreibman et al. (2015).

Indications for Use of Prelinguistic Interventions

Based on the literature reviewed by Peters-Scheffer et al. (2016), the current evidence base supports the use of PMT for children with a range of developmental delay/disability conditions. The age range for PMT intervention is chiefly young children up to 3 years of age. But children up to 8 years of age have also responded well to PMT. PMT appears well suited for use with minimally verbal children functioning at the 9–15-month level of communication development.

In terms of suitable therapeutic goals, PMT is indicated for improving outcomes on measures of intentional communication (e.g., frequency of child-initiated comments and requests, complexity of communicative acts, and increasing symbolic communication). PMT has also been associated with gains in other areas of developmental importance (e.g., improved play, increased interest in objects, and general improvement in social interaction).

In addition to there being considerable empirical support for PMT, the reviews by Dubin and Lieberman-Betz (2020) and McDaniel et al. (2022) showed that young nonverbal and minimally verbal children with autism spectrum disorder will also likely benefit from a number of other—yet conceptually and procedurally related —prelinguistic intervention programs. Prelinguistic interventions of the type reviewed by Dubin and Lieberman-Betz (2020), McDaniel et al. (2022), and Peters-Scheffer et al. (2016) are also indicated for improving joint attending skills and other language-related abilities, such as imitation, semiotic behavior, symbolic turn-taking, and verbal reciprocity. Such interventions can also be considered for situations where the child is already reliably using appropriate forms of prelinguistic behaviors that are easily recognized and have a clear meaning. For this situation, prelinguistic interventions focused on further strengthening and enhancing the child's communication abilities could potentially provide a facilitative foundation for transition to the linguistic/symbolic stage of communication development.

Contraindications for the Use of Prelinguistic Interventions

The current evidence base does not support the use of prelinguistic intervention for older participants or participants with conditions other than developmental delay/disability. This is simply because there appears to be no research that has investigated the use of prelinguistic interventions for older children and people who became nonverbal later in life due to traumatic brain injury, Alzheimer's, or amyotrophic lateral sclerosis, for example. PMT and other prelinguistic intervention programs might seem less suited to older individuals or people who had progressed past the prelinguistic stage of development prior to becoming severely disabled as would be the case for some people with traumatic brain injury for example. However, it is possible that some type of variation of currently supported prelinguistic interventions could be effective for older people and for people with other severely disabling conditions. This seems a reasonable possibility because the principles that underpin effective prelinguistic interventions (i.e., ensuring motivation, following the person's lead, and using natural social routines/interactions) would seem of some relevance to any therapeutic effort aimed at improving the adaptive functioning of people with various types of severely disabling conditions (Lancioni et al., 2012).

Prelinguistic interventions typically emphasize the importance of capturing child initiations. Such an emphasis could be contraindicated for use with children who rarely initiate. If the bulk of the instructional opportunities arise only when the child first initiates—perhaps by vocalizing while reaching for a desired item that has been placed out of reach—then fewer initiations would mean fewer instructional opportunities; a scenario that could slow or inhibit learning. Reichle (1997) noted that people with severe disability may show little inclination to initiate communicative exchanges and may therefore benefit from interventions that include more structured and therapist-initiated learning opportunities.

Prelinguistic intervention is also contraindicated when the person's prelinguistic behaviors are socially less appropriate (leading an adult's hand to a desired object) or problematic, such as when the person has a tantrum or engages in self-injury to recruit attention or request objects. In these cases, it is obviously not appropriate to focus on increasing these forms of prelinguistic behavior, even if they are functional for the person in the sense of communicating important messages to listeners. A more logical treatment approach would instead focus on replacing the socially less appropriate or problematic forms by teaching the person to use more appropriate communication forms to convey their wants and needs. For example, a child who leads an adult's hand to a needed object could be taught to instead use a manual sign to make that request. Similarly, a student who engages in self-injury when given a nonpreferred item could be taught to reject the offer and instead request an alternative using a speech-generating device (see Chap. 8) or picture-based communication strategy (see Chap. 7). In line with the above suggestions, Choi et al. (2010) successfully taught four nonverbal children with severe disabilities to use speech-generating devices or picture-based communication systems to reject the offer of wrong items (i.e., items they had not requested) and instead re-request items that they did want.

Problematic forms of prelinguistic behaviors have been successfully replaced by teaching the person to use equivalent, yet more appropriate and symbolic forms of communication (Reichle & Wacker, 2017; Sigafoos et al., 2016). Equivalent in this context means that the existing prelinguistic form and the new symbolic form targeted for intervention serve the same communication function for the person, such as both forms representing attempts to recruit attention, make requests, or indicate rejection. This approach, known as functional communication training, has a long history of demonstrated success for the treatment of problem behavior in people with severe disabilities (Durand & Moskowitz, 2019; Reichle & Wacker, 2017). Reichle and Wacker (2017) published a comprehensive review of the empirical literature on functional communication training and delineated guidelines for supporting implementation.

Functional communication training has also been successfully used to replace prelinguistic behaviors in minimally verbal children with autism spectrum disorder (Keen et al., 2001). In the Keen et al. study, the prelinguistic forms replaced were not problematic per se, but were rather seen as developmentally limiting. To advance the children's communication development, their existing prelinguistic behaviors were replaced by teaching the children to use more symbolic forms of communication. Thus, for some children, the focus of intervention might be to eventually replace prelinguistic forms—forms that are either developmentally limiting, socially less appropriate, or problematic—with more advanced and symbolic forms of communication.

Implementation Considerations

Designing a prelinguistic intervention for a specific child might begin by first identifying any potential communicative acts already present in the person's repertoire. For example, does the child currently attempt to recruit attention or request preferred items and, if so, by what means? An act (e.g., vocalizing and looking at an object) that seems to have some communication potential could then be targeted for intervention. Trembath and Iacono (2016) canvassed the use of standardized assessment of prelinguistic functioning. They reviewed standardized tools that can yield valuable information on the communicative functioning of individuals at the preintentional and prelinguistic stages of development. However, these two researchers also noted that there is a relative lack of standardized assessments for certain populations that might be candidates for some type of prelinguistic intervention, specifically minimally verbal and nonverbal adolescents and adults with autism spectrum disorder.

With respect to intervention planning, assessments aimed at identifying existing prelinguistic forms that may have communicative potential could prove useful. Brady and Keen (2016) argued that it was important for clinicians to "learn how each individual communicates" (p. 101). The underlying assumption of this quote is that even people with little communication development have the potential to communicate and may realize this potential via some type of prelinguistic behavior. Thus, individualized assessment aimed at identifying their existing communicative potential is indicated.

To this end, Sigafoos et al. (2000) developed the Inventory of Potential Communicative Acts (IPCA). The IPCA is an interview protocol designed to identify prelinguistic forms and functions. The protocol considers a range of prelinguistic behaviors (e.g., vocalizations, body movements, facial expression, gestures, gaze patterns, and problem behavior) and 10 different communicative functions (e.g., recruit attention, request, reject, comment, answer, and imitate). A recent review indicated that the IPCA was reliable and valid for identifying prelinguistic forms and functions in nonverbal and minimally verbal people with developmental disability (Sigafoos et al., 2022). Studies included in the review also used the IPCA to select prelinguistic targets, which were then successfully enhanced or replaced during intervention. More generally, these IPCA studies suggest that this type of indirect assessment approach might be helpful in identifying existing prelinguistic forms and functions in the repertories of nonverbal and minimally verbal people with severe disabilities.

Treatment intensity is no doubt an important variable that will likely influence the outcomes of prelinguistic intervention. However, total hours of intervention might not be the most important variable to consider in the quantification of treatment intensity. Rather, as noted by Warren et al. (2007), other factors—such as the number of high-quality teaching opportunities that arise within each treatment session—would likely represent important influences on child outcomes.

In addition to the density of communication opportunities, successful implementation probably depends heavily on the communicative partner's degree of responsivity, that is, the extent to which partners consistently recognize and reinforce the child's prelinguistic behaviors. When partner responsivity to the child's prelinguistic behaviors is infrequent and/or inconsistent, achieving positive outcomes may require supplemental partner responsivity training. For example, this could involve teaching the partner to realize that when the child looks at an object while vocalizing, it means that the child wants that object. Partners who are initially less responsive could, for example, be taught to (a) be alert to the child's communicative attempts, (b) acknowledge the child's request verbally (e.g., *Oh I see. You want the toy.*), and (c) respond contingently to the intended meaning of the child's prelinguistic behavior by providing reinforcing consequences (e.g., providing the child with the requested toy). A study by Tait et al. (2004), described in Box 3.2, illustrates the use of a partner responsivity intervention for enhancing or replacing prelinguistic acts.

Box 3.2 Summary of the Tait et al. (2004) Parent Responsivity Study
Tait et al. (2004) worked with the mothers of six nonverbal/minimally verbal children with cerebral palsy. Mothers were trained to be more responsive to their child's prelinguistic behaviors with the goal to either enhance or replace the prelinguistic behaviors. Intervention involved (a) creating opportunities (e.g., placing preferred items out of reach, offering a choice of two items, and calling the child's name), (b) acknowledging the child communicative attempts/initiations (e.g., *Good signing. You told me no.*), (c) prompting target responses if these did not occur during an opportunity, and (d) reinforcement (e.g., delivering requested items or interacting socially with the child when they responded to their name being called). For example, during baseline one child only made choices by directly touching one of two offered items. During intervention, this child was taught to make choices by pointing to photographs. Using photographs was considered a more advanced communication skill that would enable the child to indicate his preferences even when the available options were not physically present and directly within his reach. Another child initially made requests by looking at the presumably desired item. The mother enhanced this skill by teaching the child a three-step joint-attending sequence (i.e., look at toy, then look at the mother, and then look back at the toy). These results showed that mothers can learn to be responsive to their child's existing prelinguistic behaviors in ways that can effectively enhance or replace the child's existing prelinguistic skills.

Summary and Conclusion

Use of prelinguistic behavior may represent a viable communication strategy for some people with severe disability. Interventions based on behavior-analytic principles have been successfully applied to increase prelinguistic initiations, develop or clarify communicative intents, and establish foundational language skills (e.g., joint attending, imitation, and turn-taking). Prelinguistic intervention is primarily indicated for young children with developmental delay/disability who are functioning at the prelinguistic stage of communication development. Intervention outcomes will likely depend on partner responsivity to the person's prelinguistic behaviors as well as the quality and quantity of instructional opportunities received. Because some prelinguistic acts are developmentally limiting, less socially appropriate, and/or problematic, an alternative intervention approach focuses on replacing prelinguistic behavior by teaching the person to use more advanced/symbolic communication strategies. Strategies involving more symbolic forms of communication are considered in Chaps. 4–9.

References

Brady, N., & Keen, D. (2016). Individualized assessment of prelinguistic communication. In D. Keen, H. Meadan, N. C. Brady, & J. W. Halle (Eds.), *Prelinguistic and minimally verbal communicators on the autism spectrum* (pp. 101–119). Springer. https://doi.org/10.1007/978-981-10-0713-2_6

Choi, H., O'Reilly, M., Sigafoos, J., & Lancioni, G. (2010). Teaching requesting and rejecting sequences to four children with developmental disabilities using augmentative and alternative communication. *Research in Developmental Disabilities, 31*(2), 560–567. https://doi.org/10.1016/j.ridd.2009.12.006

Crais, E., & Ogletree, B. T. (2016). Prelinguistic communication development. In D. Keen, H. Meadan, N. C. Brady, & J. W. Halle (Eds.), *Prelinguistic and minimally verbal communicators on the autism spectrum* (pp. 9–32). Springer. https://doi.org/10.1007/978-981-10-0713-2_2

Didden, R., Korzilius, H., Smeets, E., Green, V. A., Lang, R., Lancioni, G. E., & Curfs, L. M. (2010). Communication in individuals with Rett syndrome: An assessment of forms and functions. *Journal of Developmental and Physical Disabilities, 22*(2), 105–118. https://doi.org/10.1007/s10882-009-9168-2

Dubin, A. H., & Lieberman-Betz, R. G. (2020). Naturalistic interventions to improve prelinguistic communication for children with autism spectrum disorder: A systematic review. *Review Journal of Autism and Developmental Disorders, 7*(5), 151–167. https://doi.org/10.1007/s40489-019-00184-9

Durand, V. M., & Moskowitz, L. (2019). The link between problem behavior and communication impairment in persons with developmental disabilities. *Current Developmental Disorders Reports, 6*(3), 138–144. https://doi.org/10.1007/s40474-019-00172-y

Dykstra, J. R., Boyd, B. A., Watson, L. R., Crais, E. R., & Baranek, G. T. (2012). The impact of the advancing social-communication and play (ASAP) intervention on preschoolers with autism spectrum disorder. *Autism, 16*(1), 27–44. https://doi.org/10.1177/1362361311408933

Fey, M. E., Warren, S. F., Brady, N., Finestack, L. H., Bredin-Oja, S. L., Fairchild, M., Sokol, S., & Yoder, P. J. (2006). Early effects of responsivity education/prelinguistic milieu teaching for children with developmental delays and their parents. *Journal of Speech, Language, and Hearing Research, 49*(3), 526–547. https://doi.org/10.1044/1092-4388(2006/039). Erratum in: *Journal of Speech, Language, and Hearing*, 2007, *50*(2), 549.

Frank, M. C., Braginsky, M., Yurovsky, D., & Marchman, V. A. (2017). Wordbank: An open repository for developmental vocabulary data. *Journal of Child Language, 44*(3), 677–694. https://doi.org/10.1017/S0305000916000209

Hart, B., & Risley, T. R. (1975). Incidental teaching of language in the preschool. *Journal of Applied Behavior Analysis, 8*(4), 411–420. https://doi.org/10.1901/jaba.1975.8-411

Iacono, T., Carter, M., & Hook, J. (1998). Identification of intentional communication in students with severe and multiple disabilities. *Augmentative and Alternative Communication, 14*(2), 102–114. https://doi.org/10.1080/07434619812331278246

Ingersoll, B. (2010). Brief report: Pilot randomized controlled trial of reciprocal imitation training for teaching elicited and spontaneous imitation to children with autism. *Journal of Autism and Developmental Disorders, 40*(9), 1154–1160. https://doi.org/10.1007/s10803-010-0966-2

Iverson, J. M., & Wozniak, R. H. (2016). Transitions to intentional and symbolic communication in typical development and in autism spectrum disorder. In D. Keen, H. Meadan, N. C. Brady, & J. W. Halle (Eds.), *Prelinguistic and minimally verbal communicators on the autism spectrum* (pp. 51–72). Springer. https://doi.org/10.1007/978-981-10-0713-2_4

Jeon, Y., & Lee, Y. (2023). Parental responses to prelinguistic vocalizations of very young children with typical development: A systematic review and meta-analysis. *Audiology and Speech Research, 19*(2), 91–103. https://doi.org/10.21848/asr.220074

Kasari, C., Gulsrud, A. C., Shite, S. Y., & Strawbridge, C. (2021). *The JASPER model for children with autism: Promoting joint attention, symbolic play, engagement, and regulation.* Guilford Press.

Keen, D. (2014). Prelinguistic communication. In J. Arciuli & J. Brock (Eds.), *Communication in autism* (pp. 9–28). John Benjamins Publishing.
Keen, D., Sigafoos, J., & Woodyatt, G. (2001). Replacing prelinguistic behaviors with functional communication. *Journal of Autism and Developmental Disorders, 31*(4), 385–398. https://doi.org/10.1023/1:1010612618969
Koegel, R. L., & Koegel, L. K. (Eds.). (2006). *Pivotal response treatments for autism: Communication, social, and academic development.* Paul H. Brookes Publishing Co.
Kryzak, L. A., & Jones, E. A. (2015). The effect of prompts within embedded circumscribed interests to teach initiating joint attention in children with autism spectrum disorders. *Journal of Developmental and Physical Disabilities, 27*(3), 265–284. https://doi.org/10.1007/s10882-014-9414-0
Lancioni, G. E., Singh, N. N., O'Reilly, M. F., Sigafoos, J., Belardinelli, M. O., Buonocunto, F., Sacco, V., Navarro, J., Lanzilotti, C., De Tommaso, M., Megna, M., & Badagliacca, F. (2012). Promoting adaptive behavior in persons with acquired brain injury, extensive motor and communication disabilities, and consciousness disorders. *Research in Developmental Disabilities, 33*(6), 1964–1974. https://doi.org/10.1016/j.ridd.2012.05.027
Landa, R. J., Holman, K. C., O'Neill, A. H., & Stuart, E. A. (2011). Intervention targeting development of socially synchronous engagement in toddlers with autism spectrum disorder: A randomized controlled trial. *Journal of Child Psychology and Psychiatry, 52*(1), 13–21. https://doi.org/10.1111/j.1469-7610.2010.02288.x
Liu, M., Brady, N. C., Boorom, O., Fleming, K., Yue, J., & Liu, Q. (2024). Prelinguistic communication complexity predicts expressive language in initial minimally verbal autistic children. *International Journal of Communication Disorders, 59*(1), 413–425. https://doi.org/10.1111/1460-6984-12956
Lopez, L. D., Walle, E. A., Pretzer, G. M., & Warlaumont, A. A. (2020). Adult responses to infant prelinguistic vocalizations are associated with infant vocabulary: A home observation study. *PLoS One, 15*(11), e0242232. https://doi.org/10.1371/journal.pone.0242232
McCathren, R. B. (2000). Teacher-implemented prelinguistic communication intervention. *Focus on Autism and Other Developmental Disabilities, 15*(1), 21–29. https://doi.org/10.1177/108835760001500103
McDaniel, J., Brady, N. C., & Warren, S. F. (2022). Effectiveness of responsivity intervention strategies on prelinguistic and language outcomes for children with autism spectrum disorder: A systematic review and meta-analysis of group and single case studies. *Journal of Autism and Developmental Disorders, 52*(11), 4783–4816. https://doi.org/10.1007/s10803-021-05331-y
McLean, J., & Synder-McLean, L. (1987). Form and function of communicative behaviour among persons with severe developmental disabilities. *Australia and New Zealand Journal of Developmental Disabilities, 13*(2), 83–98. https://doi.org/10.3109/13668258709023350
Peters-Scheffer, N. C., Huskens, B., Didden, R., & van der Meer, L. (2016). Prelinguistic milieu teaching. In R. Lang, T. B. Hancock, & N. N. Singh (Eds.), *Early intervention for young children with autism spectrum disorder* (pp. 151–175). Springer. https://doi.org/10.1007/978-3-319-30925-5_6
Reichle, J. (1997). Communication intervention with persons who have severe disabilities. *Journal of Special Education, 31*(1), 110–134. https://doi.org/10.1177/002246699703100110
Reichle, J., & Wacker, D. P. (2017). *Functional communication training for problem behavior.* Guilford Press.
Schreibman, L., Dawson, G., Stahmer, A. C., Landa, R., Rogers, S. J., McGee, G. G., Kasari, C., Brooke, I., Kaiser, A. P., Bruinsma, Y., McNerney, E., Wetherby, A. M., & Halladay, A. (2015). Naturalistic developmental behavioral interventions. Empirically validated treatments for autism spectrum disorder. *Journal of Autism and Developmental Disorders, 45*(8), 2411–2428. https://doi.org/10.1007/s10803-015-2407-8
Sigafoos, J., Woodyatt, G., Keen, D., Tait, K., Tucker, M., Roberts-Pennell, D., & Pittendreigh, N. (2000). Identifying potential communicative acts in children with developmental and

physical disabilities. *Communication Disorders Quarterly, 21*(2), 77–86. https://doi.org/10.1177/152574010002100202

Sigafoos, J., Arthur-Kelly, M., & Butterfield, N. (2006). *Enhancing everyday communication for children with disabilities*. Paul H. Brookes Publishing Co.

Sigafoos, J., O'Reilly, M. F., Lancioni, G. E., Carnett, A., Bravo, A., Rojeski, L., & Halle, J. W. (2016). Functional assessment of problematic forms of prelinguistic behavior. In D. Keen, H. Meadan, N. C. Brady, & J. W. Halle (Eds.), *Prelinguistic and minimally verbal communicators on the autism spectrum* (pp. 121–145). Springer. https://doi.org/10.1007/978-981-10-0713-2_7

Sigafoos, J., O'Reilly, M. F., Lancioni, G. E., Zhang, Z., & Marschik, P. B. (2022). The inventory of potential communicative acts (IPCA): Narrative review of reliability, validity, and clinical utility. *Evidence-Based Communication Assessment and Intervention, 16*(4), 105–122. https://doi.org/10.1080/17489539.2023.2255466

Tait, K., Sigafoos, J., Woodyatt, G., O'Reilly, M. F., & Lancioni, G. E. (2004). Evaluating the use of functional communication training to replace and enhance prelinguistic behaviours in six children with developmental and physical disabilities. *Disability and Rehabilitation, 26*(21/22), 1241–1254. https://doi.org/10.1080/09638280412331280253

Toth, K., Munson, J., Meltzoff, A. N., & Dawson, G. (2006). Early predictors of communication development in young children with autism spectrum disorder: Joint attention, imitation, and toy play. *Journal of Autism and Developmental Disorders, 36*(8), 993–1005. https://doi.org/10.1007/s10803-006-0137-7

Trembath, D., & Iacono, T. (2016). Standardized assessment of prelinguistic communication. In D. Keen, H. Meadan, N. C. Brady, & J. W. Halle (Eds.), *Prelinguistic and minimally verbal communicators on the autism spectrum* (pp. 75–100). Springer. https://doi.org/10.1007/978-981-10-0713-2_5

Warren, S. F., Fey, M. E., & Yoder, P. J. (2007). Differential treatment intensity research: A missing link to creating optimally effective communication interventions. *Mental Retardation and Developmental Disabilities Research Reviews, 13*(1), 70–77. https://doi.org/10.1002/mrdd.20139

Wetherby, A. M., & Woods, J. J. (2006). Early social interaction project for children with autism spectrum disorders beginning in the second year of life: A preliminary study. *Topics in Early Childhood Special Education, 26*(2), 67–82. https://doi.org/10.1177/02711214060260020201

Wetherby, A. M., Warren, S. F., & Reichle, J. (Eds.). (1998). *Transitions in prelinguistic communication*. Paul H. Brookes Publishing Co.

Zhang, V. H., Elmlinger, S. L., & Goldstein, M. H. (2024). Developmental cascades of vocal turn-taking connect prelinguistic vocalizing with early language. *Infant Behavior and Development, 75*, Article 101945. https://doi.org/10.1016/j.infbeh.2024.101945

Chapter 4
Enhancing Natural Gestures

Introduction

As noted in previous chapters, many people with severe disabilities are nonverbal or minimally verbal and are likely to remain so throughout their lives. Consequently, as noted by Reichle (1997), communication intervention for people with severe disabilities has—since about the early 1980s—been increasingly focused on teaching individuals with severe disabilities to use one or more alternative communication strategies. In Chap. 3, we reviewed interventions for strengthening prelinguistic behavior. Among the various types of prelinguistic behaviors that might be targeted for intervention, natural gestures could be viewed as having a unique status and a potential advantage over certain other prelinguistic forms (e.g., eye pointing, facial expression, and vocalizations) for individuals who are not physically limited. The main potential advantage of using natural gestures to communicate is that they tend to be more conventional and universally understood forms of body language (Cooperrider, 2019).

Natural gestures (see Table 4.1) include reaching, pointing, head nodding, and waving (Hodgdon, 2011). Many of the natural gestures described in Table 4.1 emerge early and remain communicatively useful throughout the person's life. In typically developing children, reaching, for example, tends to emerge prior to the 12 months of age, whereas communicative pointing usually develops between 18 and 24 months (Babaei et al., 2018). Negational and affirmational head nodding typically emerge between 13–15 and 16–18 months of age, respectively (Kettner & Carpendale, 2013). Imitative waving (e.g., bye-bye) emerges at about 9–16 months of age (Matsui et al., 2013).

Clough and Duff (2020) considered natural gestures to be a "fundamental component of language" (p. 1). Gesturing may often increase listeners' ability to understand communication acts that might otherwise be difficult to interpret (Goldin-Meadow & Wagner Alibali, 2013). For example, gestures may help clarify

J. Sigafoos et al., *Communication Strategies for People with Severe Disabilities*, Autism and Child Psychopathology Series,
https://doi.org/10.1007/978-3-031-83807-1_4

Table 4.1 Examples of natural gestures[a]

Natural gesture	Example/description
Head nod	Up and down head nod to indicate YES and back and forth/left to right head nod to indicate NO
Pointing	Pointing to desired object to request that object. Pointing to an object to direct listener's attention to the object
Reaching	Reaching for object
Waving	Waving hand to indicate hello or goodbye
Extending hand	Extending a hand (palm up) to receive/accept an object
Reaching out arms	Raising both arms to communicate a desire to be picked up
Shoulder shrug	Raising and lowering both shoulders to indicate *I don't know*
Showing/displaying objects	Holding out a preferred toy to show it
Cupping hand	Cupping hand behind the ear to indicate that the message was not heard
Finger to lips.	Holding index finger vertically to lips to tell another to be quiet
Thumbs up	Isolating and pointing one's thumb upwards to indicate affirmation

[a]*Note*: Based on Hodgdon (2011)

the meaning of a person's relatively unintelligible vocalizations or subtle facial expressions. If the meaning or intent of a communicative act can be clarified by a gesture, then listeners should be better able to respond in ways that will reinforce that act.

The development and use of communicative gestures may be compromised in people with severe disabilities. For example, physical impairments associated with cerebral palsy could inhibit a person's ability to point, reach, wave, and/or control yes/no head nodding. Other disability conditions might negatively impact the development and use of natural gesture less directly. Delehanty and Wetherby (2021), for example, examined the rates and types of gestures produced by young children with autism compared to typically developing children and children with developmental delay. They found significantly lower rates of gesture use by the autistic children. While all of the typically developing children used the pointing gesture, for example, only 50% of the autistic children and 74% of the developmentally delayed children did so. Head nodding, waving, and use of the thumbs-up gesture were also less frequently observed in the autistic and developmentally delayed children compared to the typically developing children.

Similar findings were reported by Balambigai et al. (2023) in a study involving five children with Down syndrome and five typically developing children. The children were matched on expressive language age, which ranged from 12 to 36 months. While the frequency of deictic gesturing (i.e., pointing, showing, giving, and requesting) was not significantly different for the two groups of children, the pattern of gesturing differed. Specifically, children with Down syndrome mainly used requesting gestures and showed less frequent use of giving, pointing, and showing. Typically developing children, in contrast, used the pointing gesture most often and request gesturing least often. The results point to a general deficit in the gestural repertoire of children with Down syndrome. However, these data should be interpreted with caution due to the relatively small number of participants studied.

In another comparative study, Glosser et al. (1998) found that patients with Alzheimer's disease showed similar rates of gesturing to healthy controls. However, their gestures tended to be less complex and more ambiguous. This was especially the case for patients having more significant linguistic impairment.

In contrast, Kim et al. (2015) reported more gesturing among adults with traumatic brain injury compared to healthy adults during a standardized word-finding test (i.e., *Test of Adolescent/Adult Word Finding*; German, 2016). Specifically, while both groups used similar amounts of iconic gesturing (e.g., swinging arms to represent playing golf), only the adults with traumatic brain injury used the pointing gesture during testing. The findings reported by Kim et al. could be specific to the testing task, which required participants to name pictures and complete sentences. It would be useful to extend this type of research by exploring the use of gesturing during everyday communication interactions between typical listeners and people with severely impaired speech due to traumatic brain injury.

When communication via speech is compromised due to disability, intervention to strengthen and encourage the use of natural gestures would seem to be a reasonable consideration for people with severe disability. Calculator and Diaz-Caneja Sela (2015) further argued that natural gestures used by people with severe disabilities often need to be enhanced to increase their transparency (i.e., guessability) and hence their effectiveness as a communication strategy. The aims of intervention targeting natural gestures could range from augmenting the person's existing (minimal) speech to providing an alternative (nonspeech) communication strategy that would, hypothetically at least, be easier for communication partners to interpret.

Several different types of natural gestures have been described in the literature. McNeill (1992), for example, defined four main types of gestures: (a) beat, (b) deictic, (c) iconic, and (d) metaphoric. The term beat gesture is usually applied to hand movements emitted by a person while that person is speaking. These hand gestures correspond to the flow or tempo of the person's speech and may help highlight or emphasize the important aspects of the spoken message. Deictic gestures, in contrast, involve pointing at some aspect of the environment, such as when a toddler points at a preferred toy to request it. However, McNeill also noted that deictic gestures cover instances such as giving directions or when referring to a past interaction or conversational thread. Iconic gestures refer to hand and arm movements that are similar in form to the action they are intended to reference, such as when a girl references the need for a drink by acting as if she were holding a cup to her mouth and drinking from it. Fourthly, metaphoric gestures are used to communicate an abstract idea, such as putting one's hands to their heart to signify love (Bernard et al., 2015).

Researchers have also made distinctions between distal, proximal, and descriptive gesturing (Guevara & Rodríguez, 2023). Distal gestures include reaching or pointing at objects without making any physical contact with the referent. In that sense, distal gestures are similar to some types of deictic gesturing as defined by McNeill (1992). In proximal or ostensive gesturing, in contrast, the person's retains contact with an object. Ostensive gesturing can involve showing and giving, such as when a child holds a toy out to show it to the parent or to offer it to a sibling. Another important type of natural gesture is the descriptive gesture. Descriptive gesturing usually involves using one's hands and arms to describe something. For example, when asked *How much cake do you want?*, the person could indicate the amount by varying the distance between their hands; wider apart for a big piece, but closer together for a smaller piece. All of these different types of natural gestures would seem to be relevant intervention targets for nonverbal and minimally verbal people with severe disabilities.

Review of Intervention Studies to Enhance Natural Gestures

There appear to be relatively few intervention studies explicitly focused on developing the natural gestures of people with severe disabilities, as distinct from the more general focus on prelinguistic behavior covered in Chap. 3. In addition, no systematic reviews appear to exist into interventions aimed at developing or enhancing natural gestures in this population. Roche et al. (2020), however, included a mini-review of three intervention studies that evaluated Calculator's *Enhanced Natural Gestures Instructional Approach* (Calculator, 2002, 2015; Calculator & Diaz-Caneja Sela, 2015). While no systematic reviews exist, there are a small number of individual studies that have sought to evoke, strengthen, and/or enhance the use of natural gestures in people with severe disabilities. Table 4.2 provides a summary of five relevant studies in this area. Table 4.2 includes the three studies by Calculator and colleagues (i.e.,Calculator, 2002, 2016; Calculator & Diaz-Caneja Sela, 2015) that were briefly summarized by Roche et al. (2020).

As indicated in Table 4.2, Calculator's *Enhanced Natural Gestures Instructional Approach* has been evaluated in three intervention studies that collectively included a total of 30 children with Angelman syndrome[1] (Calculator, 2002, 2016; Calculator & Diaz-Caneja Sela, 2015). Before reviewing each of these three studies in more detail, it will be helpful to consider the definition of enhanced natural gestures and highlight the differences between natural gestures and enhanced natural gestures as outlined by Calculator in the various descriptions of his approach. More comprehensive descriptions of Calculator's approach can be found in several publications (e.g., Calculator, 2002, 2015, 2016; Calculator & Diaz-Caneja Sela, 2015).

In terms of defining the term enhanced natural gestures, Calculator (2002, 2015) indicated four broad features of this concept. These features are that enhanced

[1]Angelman syndrome is a genetic disorder characterized by severe intellectual disability, seizures, microcephaly, and scoliosis (Clayton-Smith & Laan, 2003). There are different genetic forms of Angelman syndrome (e.g., chromosomal deletion and uniparental disomy forms). Communication is less impaired among individuals with nondeletion forms. However, most (71–90%) children with Angelman syndrome have very little or no spoken language and rely primarily on gestures to communicate (Pearson et al., 2019).

Table 4.2 Summary of intervention studies aimed at developing or enhancing natural gestures in people with severe disabilities

Study	Participants	Intervention goal(s)	Intervention procedures	Outcomes
Calculator (2002)	9 children with Angelman syndrome	To enhance child's use of distal natural gestures	Environmental arrangement, expectant delay, mand-modeling, molding/shaping, and reinforcement	Intervention was rated as acceptable, effective, reasonable, and easy to teach
Calculator and Diaz-Caneja Sela (2015)	3 children with Angelman syndrome	Foster spontaneous use of enhanced natural gestures	Modified mand-modeling/time delay, molding/shaping, and reinforcement	All 3 children acquired the targeted gestures and used them spontaneously
Calculator (2016)	18 children with Angelman syndrome	Spontaneous use of enhanced natural gestures and reduced problem behavior	Modified mand-modeling/time delay, molding/shaping, and reinforcement	Children were reported to have achieved goals and the intervention was positively rated by most parents
Ingersoll et al. (2007)	5 boys with autism spectrum disorder	To teach imitation of descriptive gestures	Following child's lead, contingent imitation, modeling, prompting, and reinforcement	Intervention increased imitation and spontaneous use of descriptive gestures
McLaughlin and Cascella (2008)	6 children with multiple disabilities	To teach distal gestures	Environmental arrangement, least-to-most prompting, and reinforcement	3 of the 6 students showed evidence of having learned a distal gesture

nature gestures (a) are physically observable actions that have a clear communicative intent, function, or purpose, (b) already exist in the person's repertoire, (c) represent refinements or variations to the person's existing natural gestures, and (d) consist primarily of distal gesturing (Calculator, 2002). However, Calculator and Diaz-Caneja Sela (2015) also indicated that some enhanced natural gestures might involve proximal gesturing. Further description of these four features is provided in Table 4.3.

In terms of the distinction between natural gestures and enhanced natural gestures, Calculator and Diaz-Caneja Sela (2015) outlined a number of pertinent points. Specifically, these researchers elaborated on the process by which enhanced natural gestures are developed from, or emerge out of, existing idiosyncratic, subtle, or natural gestures that are present in the person's repertoire. Specifically, Calculator and Diaz-Caneja Sela suggested that the transition or development from existing idiosyncratic or natural gesturing to enhanced natural gesturing requires a deliberate intervention approach. The aims of that deliberate intervention approach are to establish and/or clarify the communication intent, function, or purpose of the person's existing gestures. They also argued that existing gestures often need to be

Table 4.3 Main features of enhanced natural gestures as defined by Calculator (2002)

Feature	Description
Identified function	Enhanced natural gestures are communicative acts that serve a specific function for the person, such as being used to recruit attention, request preferred objects or assistance, and/or comment on some aspect of the environment
Already acquired	Enhanced natural gestures are communicative acts that have already been acquired and thus are present at some level of strength within the person's repertoire
Developmental potential	Enhanced natural gestures are based on existing natural gestures that have the potential to be developed in ways that will increase their guessability. Natural gestures are developed or enhanced through an intervention process that aims to increase their consistency and guessability and thus their effectiveness as a communication strategy
Distal and proximal gestures	Enhanced natural gestures typically consist of modifying an existing distal gesture, such as teaching the person to reach for and point at objects. Enhancement of proximal/ostensive gesturing might also be considered, such as teaching the child to make offers by holding up and moving items toward the intended recipient

enhanced via intervention to make the person's gesture-based communication attempts easier for listeners to recognize and interpret. In addition, for some individuals, the intervention process for enhancing natural gestures might involve replacing inappropriate forms of idiosyncratic or natural gesturing with more socially acceptable/enhanced forms. The enhancement of inappropriate forms to make them more socially acceptable is conceptually in line with the functional communication training approach that was considered in Chap. 3. For example, an existing idiosyncratic requesting gesture that involves leading a listener's hand to an object could be targeted for enhancement by teaching the child to instead use a distal (e.g., pointing) gesture.

The first study to evaluate the *Enhanced Natural Gestures Instructional Approach* (Calculator, 2002) involved nine children with Angelman syndrome. The children ranged from 3 to 10 years of age with a mean age of 7 years. All nine children were nonverbal and functioned in the severe to profound range of intellectual disability. The intervention program involved five phases. In Phase 1, parents received detailed information about the intervention program. Information was provided about the purpose of the program, which was primarily focused on ascertaining whether or not the intervention procedures were effective in "fostering more effective interactions between children with Angelman syndrome and their families at home and elsewhere" (p. 343). Parents were also taught the distinction between natural gestures and enhanced natural gestures. As part of this, it was explained that the main objective of the intervention was to modify the child's existing idiosyncratic/natural gestures to make the intended meaning of their gesturing more easily recognized (e.g., making a swimming stroke motion to request going to the pool). Parents then selected five home and/or community routines for implementing the intervention procedures (e.g., mealtimes, free play, swimming, leisure activity, and playing with the family dog). Parents were also taught, via role-play scenarios, how to collect data on the gestures used by the child.

In Phase 2, parents practiced recording the child's use of gestures in two of the five situations that they had nominated for intervention. Reliability checks were conducted to ensure parents were recording data accurately. The data collected in Phase 2 were used to identify one or two natural gestures for each of the five nominated routines. These identified gestures were then targeted in the Phase 3 intervention. Examples of targeted gestures included (a) reaching toward an object to request that object, (b) using a pushing hand gesture to reject offered items, (c) making a petting motion with the open hand to indicate a desire to play with the family dog, and (d) bringing a cupped hand to the mouth to request a drink. To enhance the identified gestures in Phase 3, parents were taught to implement four instructional tactics, specifically (a) environmental arrangement, (b) expectant delay, (c) mand-modeling, and (d) molding/shaping. Table 4.4 describes each of the four instructional tactics that parents were taught to use in the Calculator (2002) study.

In addition to these four instructional tactics, children's use of the targeted gestures produced natural reinforcement. For example, if a child used a distal reaching gesture to request an object, the parent would provide access to the object contingent upon the child producing the gesture. Similarly, if a child produced the petting motion gesture when the dog was out of reach, the parent would bring the dog within reach so the child could then play with the dog. Parents implemented these intervention procedures over a 12–14-week period (Phase 4). They also received regular feedback and guidance on implementation and data collection. In the final phase (Phase 5), parents rated program acceptability and feasibility.

Table 4.4 Four main instructional tactics for enhancing natural gestures as described by Calculator (2002)

Tactic	Description
Environmental arrangement	Arranging the environment to create the need for communicative gesturing, such as by placing desired items in view but out of reach, blocking access to a location, briefly interrupting or pausing an ongoing preferred activity, or creating a need for the child to seek assistance such as by placing snacks in a difficult to open container
Expectant delay	Looking expectantly at the child and waiting to signal the need for the child to communicate. The expectant look generally involves making eye contact, tilting one's head, leaning in toward the child, raising eyebrows, and opening the mouth while remaining silent for a period of time. The expectant delay is intended to create an opportunity and social expectation for the child to initiate a communication interaction using the targeted communicative gesture
Mand-modeling	Verbally instructing the child to produce a targeted communicative gesture
Molding/shaping	Physically assisting the child to produce the targeted communicative gesture if it does not occur in response to the environmental arrangement, expectant delay, and mand model. For example, to prompt the gesture for requesting a drink, the parent would pick up the child's dominant hand and mold it to replicate the act of holding a cup. The parent would then physically assist the child to bring the cupped hand to his or her mouth

The results of Calculator's (2002) study indicated that most parents rated the program as acceptable and reasonable/feasible. Parents also perceived the program to be effective in the sense of increasing and improving the child's ability to communicate using gestures. Parents also reported that this approach to enhancing natural gestures was something that would be easy to teach to others.

While parent ratings and perceptions of treatment acceptability and effectiveness are important, this type of data needs to be interpreted with caution. Objective data on the children's use of natural gestures prior to, and then again during and after the 12–14-week intervention period, would be necessary to determine empirically if the intervention did in fact produce meaningful changes in the children's use of the targeted gestures and whether doing so did in fact foster more effective interactions between the child and parent.

A strength of the Calculator (2002) study was that parents were supported to implement the program, which could increase ecological validity and boost the amount of intervention, as parents could conceivably incorporate learning opportunities throughout the day and across a wide range of natural routines. The fact that parental input was solicited and applied in each phase of the program might also have boosted parental buy-in and motivation to continue with the implementation of the instructional program. It is also important to note that parents were taught to use instructional tactics that have been empirically validated in numerous intervention studies involving people with severe disabilities (Brown et al., 2020; Schreibman et al., 2015). It would therefore seem reasonable to expect there could be positive outcomes for children when well-trained parents implement proven instructional tactics within regular daily routines. In summary, while the initial study by Calculator (2002) did not use an experimental design nor report objective outcome data on the children's gesture use, the results could still be seen as providing some preliminary evidence that (a) parents can identify natural gestures and (b) learn to apply well-established instructional strategies that would likely enhance their child's use of the identified natural gestures.

The second study by Calculator and Diaz-Caneja Sela (2015) involved enhancing the natural gestures of three children with Angelman syndrome. The children ranged from 9 to 10 years of age and had receptive and expressive language ages of 1–2 years, indicating severe communication impairment. Similar instructional tactics to those used by Calculator (2002) were implemented, except that environmental arrangement was not used and the expectant delay tactic was combined with mand-modeling, rather than being used as separate procedures. Another change was the use of nonspecific verbal prompts (e.g., *What do you want?*) prior to using the time delay/mand-modeling procedure or the molding/shaping technique. In addition, this study was implemented by teaching staff, rather than parents, and the study was conducted in the children's classroom, rather than the home environment.

Over the 12-week intervention period of the Calculator and Diaz-Caneja Sela (2015) study, objective-observational data were collected on each child's spontaneous versus nonspontaneous (prompted) use of enhanced natural gestures. A spontaneous gesture was recorded when the child produced the gesture without staff prompting (i.e., when staff had not used any nonspecific verbal prompts, mand-models, or molding/shaping). Nonspontaneous gestures, in contrast, were recorded if the gesture occurred after prompting. The results showed increases in the spontaneous use of gestures and decreased need for prompting from week 1 to week 12. Such trends were evidenced for all three children. For example, in week 1, one child (Sonia) was observed to have produced 51 nonspontaneous gestures and only 5 spontaneous gestures. In week 12, however, she produced fewer nonspontaneous (n = 13) gestures and many more spontaneous gestures (n = 35).

The increases reported by Calculator and Diaz-Caneja Sela (2015) over the 12 weeks of their program provide some evidence to support the use of the *Enhanced Natural Gestures Instructional Approach* for increasing spontaneous use of enhanced natural gestures by the three participating children with Angelman syndrome. These data also suggest that the *Enhanced Natural Gestures Instructional Approach* can be effectively implemented by school staff in classroom settings. However, the results need to be interpreted with caution due to the use of a pre-experimental (i.e., teaching-only) design. The design did not include any nonteaching baselines or other control condition that would enable one to confidently assert that the observed increases in spontaneous gesturing over the 12-week program were due to staff implementation of the instructional procedures. It is possible, for example, that the changes in the children's ratios of spontaneous to nonspontaneous gesturing were related to maturation, changes in motivational levels, and/or changes in the number and type of communication opportunities arising in the classroom.

Further supporting evidence for the potential value of the *Enhanced Natural Gestures Instructional Approach* was provided in a third study involving 18 children with Angelman syndrome (Calculator, 2016). The children ranged from about 3–18 years of age and had expressive language ages indicative of severe communication impairment. Parents set goals for their child and quantified goal attainment on a 5-point scale, ranging from −2 (worst expected outcome) to +2 (best expected outcome). An example of a best expected outcome was: "Uses 75–100% of enhanced natural gestures spontaneously or in response to non-specific verbal prompts, at least once each day, without the need for mand-modeling or molding/shaping" (p. 4). An example of a worst expected outcome was: "Always requires either a mand-model or molding/shaping prompt to use enhanced natural gestures; never uses any enhanced natural gestures spontaneously or in response to non-specific verbal prompts" (p. 4). A unique feature of this study was that parents received a manual describing the *Enhanced Natural Gestures Instructional Approach* and essentially followed the manual in a self-instructional process, although parents were also supported by a consultant speech-language pathologist. The manual defined enhanced natural gestures, the associated assessment and intervention procedures, and procedures for evaluating the program using goal attainment scaling (Kiresuk & Sherman, 1968). At the end of the 10-week program, most children were rated as having met or exceeded expectations. Parents' perceptions of the program were favorable, and they also reported no major implementation problems. Based on these results, the author concluded that enhanced natural gestures may "represent a viable method of communication for many individuals with Angelman syndrome" (p. 1). However, the author also acknowledged that his design was pre-experimental and therefore any "definitive statements pertaining to program efficacy are premature" (p. 3).

Collectively, the results of the three studies that have evaluated the *Enhanced Natural Gestures Instructional Approach* (Calculator, 2002, 2016; Calculator & Diaz-Caneja Sela, 2015) are limited in the sense that the reported improvements cannot be unequivocally attributed to implementation of the program due to the use of pre-experimental designs. Still, given the results reported so far, there would seem to be sufficient promise in this approach to warrant additional research using more rigorous experimental designs. While future research is called for, there would seem to be little possible harm in recommending Calculator's *Enhanced Natural Gestures Instructional Approach*, given that it aims to enhance existing gestures that have a clear communicative potential via the implementation of well-established instructional tactics.

In addition to enhancing natural gestures, researchers have also evaluated interventions aimed at directly teaching specific new forms of natural gesturing. Along these lines, the study by Ingersoll et al. (2007) is a good example of this type of intervention research. Specifically, the aim of the Ingersoll et al. study was to teach correct imitation of descriptive gesturing. Participants were five young boys with autism spectrum disorder, who ranged from 34 to 49 months of age. Four of these boys were rated as having severe autism symptoms and the other child was considered to have mild/moderate autism. Assessments revealed that the children had cognitive delays ranging from 12–21 months and language delays of 13–24 months.

The intervention program developed by Ingersoll et al. (2007) focused on teaching the children to imitate descriptive gestures modeled led by the therapist. Data were also collected on the children's spontaneous use of descriptive gestures. The types of descriptive gestures targeted for training included (a) a palms-up response to signify a request for information (*Where is it?*), (b) hands-on-face to indicate an affective response (*Oh no!*), (c) gestures to describe objects (e.g., arms stretched out and moved like airplane wings), and (d) gestures to communicate attributes and actions, such as the concept *big* or the action *spin*.

A multicomponent intervention package, referred to as Reciprocal Imitation Training, was implemented. The training protocol included contingent imitation and linguistic mapping,[2] following the child's lead, physical prompting, and reinforcement. Intervention sessions of 20-min duration occurred 2 days per week for 10 weeks. Sessions occurred in a small treatment room during free play with the therapist. To teach the targeted gestures, the therapist would model a specific gesture (e.g., finger to lips) while making a verbal comment (e.g., *Shh, the baby's sleeping.*). Models for the child to imitate were provided by the therapist about once per minute. A gesture could be modeled up to three times and correct imitation by the child resulted in praise and continuation of play. If a correct response did not occur,

[2] Contingent imitation involved the therapist imitating the child's behavior, including the child's actions and vocalizations. Linguistic mapping refers to the therapist making comments about the ongoing activity.

the therapist physically prompted the gesture and reinforced the prompted response with praise.

The effects of these intervention procedures were evaluated in a multiple baseline across participants' design. Prior to introducing the intervention package, children received from 7 to 14 baseline sessions during which gestures were modeled but not directly taught. Gesture imitation rarely occurred during baseline. With intervention, gesture imitation increased to varying levels—from 10 to 20% (for one participant) and from 40 to 50% (for another participant)—by the end of the 10-week intervention phase. Importantly, clear and consistent increases in spontaneous use of gestures were observed for three of the five children. Maintenance of the intervention gains made by children was assessed at a 1-month follow-up. At follow-up, all the children were performing at levels below that achieved during their intervention, but they were still imitating at levels that were generally above the low levels observed during baseline.

The results of Ingersoll et al.'s (2007) study point to the feasibility of teaching descriptive gestures to children with severe autism using a naturalistic/play-based intervention approach, similar to the types of naturalistic developmental behavioral interventions for prelinguistic skills that were reviewed in Chap. 3. Overall, the results suggest that, with about 20 h of Reciprocal Imitation Training, it would be reasonable to expect that children with severe autism could acquire and spontaneously use a number of different descriptive gestures.

The fifth and final study summarized in Table 4.2 set out to teach the use of a pointing gesture to six (8–13-year-old) nonverbal students with multiple disabilities (McLaughlin & Cascella, 2008). The children had severe or moderate–severe intellectual disability and additional conditions, such as Angelman syndrome, attention-deficit hyperactivity disorder, cerebral palsy, seizure disorder, and/or vision impairment. An initial assessment indicated that none of the six participants were using distal gestures, such as pointing. In the next phase, to teach distal gesturing, the students were presented with four types of response/gesture opportunities: (a) wind-up toys placed out of reach, (b) a remote-controlled car was activated in reach of the child, (c) mechanical toy animal activated in reach of the child, and (d) choice between a preferred and nonpreferred item. Opportunities were embedded into three play sessions of 30–40 min each. Across the three sessions, each child received 12 total opportunities to use the targeted distal gesture (i.e., four opportunities per session). A least-to-most prompting strategy was implemented to teach distal gesturing. For example, the researcher would activate the wind-up toy and place it out of the child's reach. If the child did not produce the gesture (i.e., pointing at the toy), the researcher provided a verbal prompt. If the verbal prompt was not successful in recruiting the gesture from the child, the researcher then added a modeling prompt (i.e., pointing to the toy) while repeating the verbal prompt (e.g., *Point to the toy*). If that level of prompting was still not successful in evoking the distal gesture from the child, the researcher added increasing levels of physical prompting (tapping the child's arm, using hand-over-hand guidance). After prompting, the toy was reactivated, which was assumed to represent a form of natural reinforcement for the child's distal gesture.

The overall results of this study were mixed. Three of the six students failed to show any evidence of having learned the distal gesture. The other participants showed some evidence of learning in that they produced a distal gesture in 3–4 of their 12 total opportunities. These gains could be seen as relatively modest, which could reflect the fact that each child received only 12 learning opportunities in total. Still, the fact that learning was evident for half the sample in a mere 12 trials suggests that a combination of environmental arrangement, least-to-most prompting, and natural reinforcement might be an effective way of teaching distal gesturing to nonverbal students with severe/multiple disabilities. However, most such children would likely require many more learning opportunities to acquire distal gestures of this type.

Indications for the Use of Natural Gestures

Development and enhancement of natural gestures may represent a viable approach for improving the communication for people with severe disabilities. Natural gestures may represent an effective communication strategy because these acts tend to be fairly universally used and readily understood within a given cultural context (Cooperrider, 2019). They could also be seen as a functional and developmentally appropriate habilitative goal because natural gesturing tends to emerge early and will likely remain useful to the person throughout their life.

For people with severe disability, use of natural gestures may represent an important compensatory form of communication when speech development is minimal. When speech is severely impaired, as when the person is essentially nonverbal, the use of natural gestures may represent an important and perhaps even a primary mode of communication. Even when other augmentative and alternative communication modes are taught, such as use of manual signing (Chap. 5) or use of speech-generating devices (Chap. 8), development and enhancement of natural gestures could be indicated as they can provide the person with an additional/supplemental communication strategy. For example, candidates for learning to use formal manual signs or speech-generating devices might find it easier and more effective to use natural gestures (e.g., reaching, pointing, waving, showing, and affirmative head nodding) in certain situations, such as when needing to communicate a simple idea (e.g., *Yes* or *I want that.*) to a listener unfamiliar with sign language or less experienced in deciphering the digitized speech output of a speech-generating device. Iacono (2019) noted advantages of teaching multiple augmentative and alternative communication strategies (e.g., manual signing, picture-exchange, and speech-generating devices) to people with complex communication needs. Natural gestures could therefore be indicated for inclusion as part of any such multimodal approach to communication intervention for people with severe disabilities. In fact, natural gestures might be seen as a critical component of communication intervention as they present a more robust and natural supplement to any communication strategy—evidenced by the fact that typically developing people use gestures throughout their lives.

The *Enhanced Natural Gestures Instructional Approach* (Calculator, 2002, 2016; Calculator & Diaz-Caneja Sela, 2015) has so far been used only with children and adolescents with Angelman syndrome. However, there is no logical reason why the approach would not also be applicable to people with similarly severe disabilities. The *Enhanced Natural Gestures Instructional Approach* is primarily indicated for enhancing the clarity and consistency of distal gestures. It is therefore indicated for people with existing idiosyncratic or natural forms of distal gesturing that occur either too infrequently or inconsistently and/or when the meaning of the gesture is not sufficiently clear.

In cases where the person has not yet acquired an effective range of natural gestures, intervention aimed at directly teaching new forms of natural gestures is indicated. To this end, the systematic instructional approaches described by Ingersoll et al. (2007) and McLaughlin and Cascella (2008) show promise for teaching spontaneous use of descriptive and distal gesturing to children with autism and multiple disabilities. These same instructional tactics might also prove effective in teaching other types of natural gestures. However, additional research is needed to confirm this possibility. There is also a need for additional intervention research to establish indications for other populations. For example, given that patients with Alzheimer's disease tend to have less complex and more ambiguous gestures (Glosser et al., 1998), there could be some potential benefit to an enhancement-focused intervention approach for this population.

Contraindications for the Use of Natural Gestures

There seem to be no major contraindications to the development and/or enhancement of natural gestures as a communication strategy for people with severe disabilities. Calculator (2002, 2015), however, explained that if an existing natural gesture was socially inappropriate, then intervention should aim to enhance that gesture in ways that would make it more conventional and socially acceptable. For example, some children might forcibly and aggressively push away unwanted objects. For these situations, the priority could be to enhance this natural reject gesture by teaching the child to hold out their arm with their palm facing out to indicate *Stop*. Technically, in the above example, an existing proximal gesture (i.e., making direct contact to push an item away) is enhanced (or replaced) by developing a functionally equivalent distal gesture (i.e., extending one's arm and palm outward as the nonpreferred object is offered). Functional communication training (see Chap. 3) would be recommended in such situations, and the aim would be to replace unacceptable responses with more appropriate responses.

Implementation Considerations

A number of factors are important to consider when designing an intervention to develop and enhance the use of natural gestures as a communication strategy for people with severe disabilities. Factors to consider include (a) selection of natural gestures, (b) correct application of the intervention procedures, and (c) scheduling sufficient amounts of intervention. In terms of selecting natural gestures, Calculator (2002, 2015) emphasized the importance of undertaking assessments to document the person's existing range of gestures. Assessment should include direct and repeated observations of the person's gestural responses to various types of structured communication opportunities, such as when a preferred item is placed out of reach, when the person needs help with a task, and when nonpreferred objects are offered. During each observation trial, data should be collected on the specific form or topography of any gestures emitted and the likely purpose or intent of the emitted gestures. Stakeholders would then review this data to select existing gestures that need to be enhanced to make them more fluent and understandable.

Initial assessment data may also indicate that a person is not using any natural gesture at all. In other cases, the person might be using some natural gestures, but infrequently or only when prompted to do so. In these cases, intervention could focus on directly teaching and increasing spontaneous use of natural gestures, as was illustrated in the studies by Ingersoll et al. (2007) and McLaughlin and Cascella (2008).

Successful intervention outcomes will likely depend on the extent to which the intervention procedures are implemented with fidelity. Calculator (2002, 2016) and Calculator and Diaz-Caneja Sela (2015), for example, provided extensive training and regular feedback to parents and teaching staff to ensure correct implementation of the *Enhanced Natural Gestures Instructional Approach.* Similarly, correct use of the types of instructional procedures described by Ingersoll et al. (2007) and McLaughlin and Cascella (2008) may also require personnel with expertise and competencies related to (a) objectively defining one or more discrete natural gestures for intervention, (b) creating multiple, structured teaching opportunities, (c) using one or more response prompts to reliably evoke the targeted gesture during each opportunity, (d) fading response prompts systematically to promote spontaneous use of natural gestures, and (e) providing natural reinforcement to strengthen and maintain the person's spontaneous use of their newly acquired natural gestures.

With respect to scheduling intervention sessions, data reviewed in this chapter suggest that positive outcomes will likely require consistent (daily) intervention sessions over a protracted period of time (e.g., 10–12 weeks). Brief, lower-intensity interventions—such as the 12-opportunity program run by McLaughlin and Cascella (2008)—would, in contrast, likely produce the much more modest outcomes reported by these two researchers. Finally, assessing and teaching these gestures within natural contexts, and supporting key individuals within those contexts (e.g., parents and teachers), to teach and reinforce natural gestures may promote maintenance and generalization of these gestures (Stokes & Baer, 1977).

Summary and Conclusion

Use of natural gestures is a potentially viable and effective communication strategy for people with severe disabilities. The results of the studies reviewed in this chapter suggest that natural gestures can be taught and enhanced using naturalistic, play-based approaches that incorporate well-established systematic instructional procedures. Studies have successfully taught spontaneous use of descriptive natural gestures to children with autism spectrum disorder (Ingersoll et al., 2007) and increased distal gesturing in children with severe/multiple disability (McLaughlin & Cascella, 2008). A specific manualized program developed by Calculator and his colleague (Calculator, 2002, 2016; Calculator & Diaz-Caneja Sela, 2015) also appears promising for enhancing natural gestures in children and adolescents with Angelman syndrome.

Development and enhancement of natural gestures are widely indicated with few contraindications. However, additional research is needed to establish the utility of similar intervention approaches for developing a wider range of gesture types in people with other severe disability conditions. Factors that need to be considered for intervention design include (a) selection of target gestures, (b) adherence to intervention protocols, and (c) the amount and duration (i.e., intensity) of intervention.

Development and enhancement of natural gestures may represent a possible strategy for augmenting minimal speech. Increasing natural gestures may also provide an alternative communication strategy for nonverbal individuals. Natural gesture can also be incorporated within a larger multimodal augmentative and alternative communication system.

References

Babaei, Z., Zarifian, T., Ashtari, A., Bakhshi, E., & Ebrahimpour, M. (2018). A look at the normal development of pointing and reaching gestures in 12-16-month-old Farsi-speaking children: A longitudinal study. *Iranian Journal of Child Neurology, 12*(4), 127–139.

Balambigai, N., Chittathur, U. R., Kanagamuthu, P., & Ganesh, J. (2023). Investigating the use of gestures among children with down syndrome in India. *Journal of Modern Rehabilitation, 17*(4), 394–402. https://doi.org/10.18502/jmr.v17i4.13887

Bernard, J. A., Millman, Z. B., & Mittal, V. A. (2015). Beat and metaphoric gestures are differentially associated with regional cerebellar and cortical volumes. *Human Brain Mapping, 36*(1), 4016–4030. https://doi.org/10.1002/hbm.22894

Brown, F., McDonnell, J., & Snell, M. (2020). *Instruction of students with severe disabilities* (9th ed.). Pearson.

Calculator, S. N. (2002). Use of enhanced natural gestures to foster interactions between children with Angelman syndrome and their parents. *American Journal of Speech-Language Pathology, 11*(4), 340–355. https://doi.org/10.1044/1058-0360(2002/039)

Calculator, S. N. (2015). Enhanced natural gestures: A self-administered program for teaching communication behaviors to individuals with Angelman syndrome. In S. N. Calculator (Ed.), *Angelman syndrome: Communication, educational and related considerations* (pp. 192–216). Bentham Science Publishers. https://doi.org/10.2174/9781681081168115010l

Calculator, S. (2016). Description and evaluation of a home-based parent-administered program for teaching enhanced natural gestures to individuals with Angelman syndrome. *American Journal of Speech-Language Pathology, 25*(1), 1–13. https://doi.org/10.1044/2015_AJSLP-15-0017
Calculator, S., & Diaz-Caneja Sela, P. (2015). Overview of the enhanced natural gestures instructional approach and illustration of its use with three students with Angelman syndrome. *Journal of Applied Research in Intellectual Disabilities, 28*(2), 145–158. https://doi.org/10.1111/jar.12110
Clayton-Smith, J., & Laan, L. (2003). Angelman syndrome: A review of the clinical and genetics aspects. *Journal of Medical Genetics, 40*(2), 87–95. https://doi.org/10.1136/jmg.40.2.87
Clough, S., & Duff, M. C. (2020). The role of gesture in communication and cognition: Implications for understanding and treating neurogenic communication disorders. *Frontiers in Human Neuroscience, 14*(323). https://doi.org/10.3389/fnhum.2020.00323
Cooperrider, K. (2019). Universals and diversity in gesture research past, present, and future. *Gesture, 18*(2–3), 209–238. https://doi.org/10.1075/gest.19011.coo
Delehanty, A. D., & Wetherby, A. M. (2021). Rate of communicative gestures and developmental outcomes in toddlers with and without autism spectrum disorder during a home observation. *American Journal of Speech-Language Pathology, 30*(2), 649–662. https://doi.org/10.1044/2020_AJSLP-19-00206
German, D. J. (2016). *TAWF-2: Test of adolescent/adult word finding* (2nd ed.). Pro-Ed.
Glosser, G., Wiley, M. J., & Barnoski, E. J. (1998). Gestural communication in Alzheimer's disease *Journal of Clinical and Experimental Neuropsychology 20*(1) 1–13. https://doi.org/10.1076/jcen.20.1.1.1484
Goldin-Meadow, S., & Wagner Alibali, M. (2013). Gesture's role in speaking, learning, and creating language. *Annual Review of Psychology, 64*, 257–283. https://doi.org/10.1146/annurev-psych-113011-143802
Guevara, I., & Rodríguez, C. (2023). Developing communication through objects: Ostensive gestures as the first gestures in children's development. *Developmental Review, 68*, 1–26. https://doi.org/10.1016/j.dr.2023.101076
Hodgdon, L. A. (2011). *Visual strategies for improving communication: Practical supports for autism spectrum disorders* (3rd ed.). Quirk Roberts Publishing.
Iacono, T. (2019). An exploration of multimodality in augmentative and alternative communication. *Journal of Clinical Practice in Speech-Language Pathology, 29*(3), 126–130. https://doi.org/10.1080/22087168.2019.12370265
Ingersoll, B., Lewis, E., & Kroman, E. (2007) Teaching the imitation and spontaneous use of descriptive gestures in young children with autism using a naturalistic behavioral intervention *Journal of Autism and Developmental Disorders 37*(8) 1446–1456. https://doi.org/10.1007/s10803-006-0221-z
Kettner, V. A., & Carpendale, J. I. M. (2013). Developing gestures for *no* and *yes*: Head shaking and nodding in infancy. *Gesture, 13*(2), 193–209. https://doi.org/10.1075/gest.13.2.04ket
Kim, M. J., Stierwalt, J. A. G., LaPointe, L. L., & Bourgeois, M. S. (2015). The use of gestures following traumatic brain injury: A preliminary analysis. *Aphasiology, 26*(6), 665–684. https://doi.org/10.1080/02687038.2014.976536
Kiresuk, T., & Sherman, R. (1968). Goal attainment scaling: A general method for evaluating comprehensive community mental health programs. *Community Mental Health Journal, 4*(6), 443–453. https://doi.org/10.1007/BF01530764
Matsui, G., Ohtoshi, T., & Takada, S. (2013). Imitation of 'bye-bye' in very low-birthweight infants. *Pediatrics International, 55*(5), 561–565. https://doi.org/10.1111/ped.12160
McLaughlin, K., & Cascella, P. W. (2008). Eliciting a distal gesture via dynamic assessment among students with moderate to severe intellectual disability *Communication Disorders Quarterly 29*(2) 75–81. https://doi.org/10.1177/1525740107311821
McNeill, D. (1992). *Hand and mind: What gestures reveal about thought*. University of Chicago Press.

Pearson, E., Wilde, L., Heald, M., Royston, R., & Oliver, C. (2019). Communication in Angelman syndrome: A scoping review. *Developmental Medicine and Child Neurology, 61*(11), 1266–1274. https://doi.org/10.1111/dmcn.14257

Reichle, J. (1997). Communication intervention with persons who have severe disabilities. *Journal of Special Education, 31*(1), 110–134. https://doi.org/10.1177/002246699703100110

Roche, L., Sigafoos, J., & Trembath, D. (2020). Augmentative and alternative communication intervention for people with Angelman syndrome: A systematic review. *Current Developmental Disorders Reports, 7*(1), 28–34. https://doi.org/10.1007/s40474-020-00187-w

Schreibman, L., Dawson, G., Stahmer, A. C., Landa, R., Rogers, S. J., McGee, G. G., Kasari, C., Brooke, I., Kaiser, A. P., Bruinsma, Y., McNerney, E., Wetherby, A. M., & Halladay, A. (2015). Naturalistic developmental behavioral interventions. Empirically validated treatments for autism spectrum disorder. *Journal of Autism and Developmental Disorders, 45*(8), 2411–2428. https://doi.org/10.1007/s10803-015-2407-8

Stokes, T. F., & Baer, D. M. (1977). An implicit technology of generalization. *Journal of Applied Behavior Analysis, 10*(2), 349–367. https://doi.org/10.1901/jaba.1977.10-349

Chapter 5
Teaching Manual Signs

Introduction

Within the field of augmentative and alternative communication, a distinction is made between aided and unaided communication strategies (Beukelman & Light, 2020; Crowe et al., 2022; Fuller & Pampoulou, 2022; Ganz, 2014; Syriopoulou-Delli & Eleni, 2022). Aided communication strategies make use of some type of external aid or equipment. Common examples of aided communication strategies include (a) exchanging pictures or photographs, (b) selecting symbols or letters from a picture board or alphabet board, (c) pointing to or touching miniature or tangible objects that function as communication symbols, and (d) selecting communication symbols/icons from the screen of a computer-based speech-generating device. Research related to aided communication strategies is reviewed in Chaps. 6–9.

Unaided communication strategies, in contrast, do not require any external materials or equipment. Spoken language is perhaps the most obvious and commonly understood and used mode of unaided communication. But for people with severe disabilities who cannot rely on speech to meet their everyday communication needs, other unaided strategies can be considered. Some of these other unaided communication strategies include the use of prelinguistic behavior (Chap. 3) and natural gestures (Chap. 4). Manual signing, which is the topic of the present chapter, is an additional type of unaided communication strategy that is frequently considered for nonverbal and minimally verbal people with severe disabilities.

Manual signing can be viewed as a way of transmitting messages using one's hands, arms, and fingers. In this respect, a manual sign can be topographically similar to certain prelinguistic acts and natural gestures. However, unlike prelinguistic acts and natural gestures, manual signs are generally drawn from more formalized

J. Sigafoos et al., *Communication Strategies for People with Severe Disabilities*, Autism and Child Psychopathology Series,
https://doi.org/10.1007/978-3-031-83807-1_5

linguistic (sign language) systems. American Sign Language, for example, is a formal manual language used by the Deaf in Canada and the United States (Stewart & Stewart, 2021). American Sign Language includes individual signs and sign combinations representing nouns, verbs, and concepts (see Fig. 5.1 for examples). American Sign Language also has a standardized system of finger spelling with various finger/hand configurations representing different letters of the alphabet.

For the Deaf in Canada and the United States, American Sign Language is the linguistic equivalent of a formal spoken language. Internationally, there are hundreds of formal sign languages for the Deaf. The Deaf in Australia, for example, use Auslan (Johnston & Schembri, 2007), while British Sign Language is the language of the Deaf in the United Kingdom (Deuchar, 2013). These formal sign languages are not merely signed equivalents of spoken language, but rather have their own grammatical structure and syntax, as well as unique forms and lexicon.

In communication interventions for people with severe disabilities, the targeting of manual sign-based strategies does not necessarily mean that the person has to be taught a formal sign language with all its grammatical complexities. Rather, the person might be taught to use some individual manual signs and manual sign combinations. And, while the specific target signs could be selected from the lexicon of a formal sign language or sign system, they might also be selected from the many other less formal, more limited, and/or more simplified sign systems that exist (Bonvillian et al., 2020; Grove & Walker, 1990; Meuris et al., 2014).

Key word signing (Grove & Dockrell, 2000), for example, is a relatively less formalized approach to the teaching of manual signing compared to an intervention targeting fluency in say American Sign Language or Auslan. With a key word approach, the main concept of a spoken sentence is emphasized by simultaneous production of a corresponding manual sign (Grove & Dockrell, 2000). Meuris et al. (2014) noted that the actual manual signs that might be used in a key word signing approach could be selected from "any sign language or sign system" (p. 991). Key word signing has also been hypothesized as a possible means of supporting speech and language development for people with language delay (Meuris et al., 2014). Thus, for some people, key word signing could represent their primary

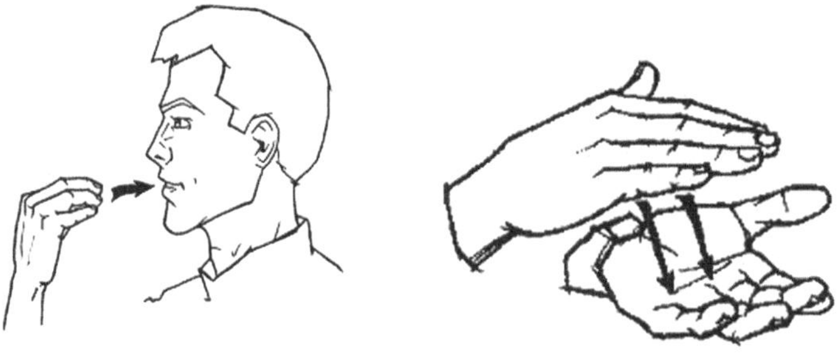

Fig. 5.1 American Sign Language: manual signs for EAT and SCHOOL

communication strategy. But for others it may represent a temporary aid to facilitate and accelerate speech and language development (Meuris et al., 2014).

Somewhat akin to key word signing is the approach known as simultaneous or total communication (Carr, 1979). In a simultaneous or total communication approach, the interventionist models the use of both sign and corresponding speech. For example, an interventionist could simultaneously say and sign the word DRINK or HELP during instructional opportunities, such as opportunities aimed at teaching the person to ask for a drink or ask for help with difficult tasks. For some minimally verbal individuals, the simultaneous combination of speech and sign might not only lead to acquisition of the targeted manual signs, but could also facilitate that person's natural speech production (Goldstein, 2002; Pattison & Robertson, 2016; Remington & Clarke, 1983). Simultaneous communication might also be explored for its potential benefit in supporting receptive communication (e.g., increased comprehension of both speech and manual signs).

Review of Intervention Studies on Teaching Manual Signs

An extensive research literature on teaching manual signing to people with severe disabilities has developed over the past several decades. To illustrate the nature and range of research in this area, Table 5.1 summarizes 23 intervention studies aimed at teaching, increasing, and/or otherwise enhancing the use of manual signing by people with different types of severely disabling conditions. Studies from different decades were selected to illustrate the range of intervention goals pursued and the range of instructional tactics that have been successfully used in teaching, increasing, and/or enhancing the use of manual signing as a communication strategy for people with severe disabilities. The studies in Table 5.1 are summarized in terms of participants, intervention goals, intervention procedures, and outcomes. In the following narrative overview, a selection of studies from Table 5.1 are grouped according to participant population, curriculum orientation, and general intervention approach.

Studies Involving Nonverbal and Minimally Verbal Autistic Children

The 1978 study by Carr et al. (summarized in the first row of Table 5.1) appears to be the first systematic and experimentally controlled attempt at teaching manual signing to nonverbal children with autism. In this study, four nonverbal autistic children (10–15 years of age) were successfully taught to produce manual signs representing five different foods and beverages (i.e., apple, banana, candy, cookie, and milk). The teaching procedures involved the therapist offering one of the objects

Table 5.1 Summary of 23 intervention studies on teaching and increasing manual sign use among people with severe disabilities

Study	Participants	Intervention goal(s)	Intervention procedures	Outcomes
Carr et al. (1978)	4 nonverbal children with autism (aged 10–15 years)	Produce the correct manual sign for each of five items when shown the item	Present object plus verbal label, physical prompting, prompt fading, and reinforcement	Children required from 948, to 7669 trials to achieve mastery.
Carr and Kologinsky (1983)	6 autistic children (aged 9–14 years)	Increase spontaneous use of manual signed request	Adult approach, imitative prompting, prompt fading, and reinforcement	Spontaneous requesting increased
Carr et al. (1987)	4 nonverbal autistic boys (aged 11–16 years)	Generalized use of action-object sign combinations	Physical prompting, prompt fading, and reinforcement	Generalized use of sign combinations required from 1208 to 11,155 trials
Kleinert and Gast (1981)	31-year-old nonverbal man with cerebral palsy and severe/profound hearing impairment	To teach expressive use and assess receptive understanding of six work-related manual signs	Verbal and visual cueing, modeling, 0-s and 4-s time delay, error correction, and reinforcement	Participant acquired expressive use of all six signs within 150 training trials and also showed correct comprehension of signs
Coelho and Duffy (1985)	61-year-old male with nonfluent aphasia due to stroke	Acquisition of 90 manual signs representing nouns, verbs, and adjectives	A three-stage imitation, recognition and production training protocol was followed	Acquired 73 of the 90 signs, but did not use the acquired signs spontaneously
Coelho and Duffy (1986)	12 aphasic adults (aged 30–67 years)	To assess the influence of iconicity, motor complexity, and linguistic function on acquisition of manual signs	Imitation, Recognition, and Production training on 37 manual signs as per Coelho and Duffy (1985)	Acquisition was better for more iconic and less motorically complex signs representing verbs
Coelho (1987)	21-year-old female with aphasia and verbal apraxia due to traumatic brain injury	To teach manual sign production related to wants and needs	Imitation, Recognition, and Production training as per Coelho and Duffy (1985, 1986)	47 signs learned in 5 months. Signs not used spontaneously

(continued)

Table 5.1 (continued)

Study	Participants	Intervention goal(s)	Intervention procedures	Outcomes
Coelho and Duffy (1987)	12 aphasic adults (aged 30–67 years)	To investigate the relation between severity of aphasia and acquisition of manual signs	Imitation, Recognition, and Production training on 37 manual signs as per Coelho and Duffy (1985, 1986)	Participants acquired 20–100% of signs and severity of aphasia negatively affected acquisition
Duker and Michielsen (1983)	3 nonverbal children (aged 8–16 years) with severe intellectual disability	To teach generalized use of 3–4 manual signs in response to verbal instructions	Verbal instruction, object presentation, modeling, faded physical assistance (i.e., graduated guidance), and reinforcement	Targeted signs were acquired in 5–28 sessions. Correct signing generalized across people and settings
Duker and Morsink (1984)	4 individuals (aged 8–23 years) with severe intellectual disability	To teach generalized use of 3–4 manual signs in response to verbal instructions or visual cues	Verbal instruction, object presentation, modeling, faded physical assistance (i.e., graduated guidance), and reinforcement	Targeted signs were acquired in 4–23 sessions. Correct signing generalized across settings
Seys et al. (1990)	9 individuals (aged 9–26 years) with intellectual disability	To increase spontaneous use of manually signed requests	Staff were taught to create increased signing opportunities, and to prompt and reinforce signed requests	Mean number of spontaneous signed requests increased with intervention for 8 of the 9 participants. Gains were maintained at follow-up for 7 of the 9 participants
Duker et al. (1991)	14 individuals (aged 11–35 years) with severe–profound intellectual disability and self-injurious behavior	To examine effects of teaching manual signed requests on self-injury with at least 10 signs targeted per person	Time delay, most-to-least prompting, verbal cueing (*what do you want*), and reinforcement. SIB followed by 2 min of verbal and physical prompting of signing	Signed requesting increased and self-injury decreased for all but one participant
Duker and van Lent (1991)	6 individuals (aged 12–30 years) with severe–profound intellectual disability	To increase the number of different manual signs used spontaneously	Reinforcement was provided for signs used less frequency and reinforcement was withheld for the 2–3 signs used most frequently	43% increase in the number of different signs emitted during intervention versus baseline sessions

(continued)

Table 5.1 (continued)

Study	Participants	Intervention goal(s)	Intervention procedures	Outcomes
Duker et al. (1993)	4 people (aged 14–31 years) with severe–profound intellectual disability	To teach participants to reject items that did not match their prior signed request	Verbal and physical prompting, error correction/response interruption, response repetition, and reinforcement	With training, the percentage of trials in which nonmatching items were rejected increased from baseline
Duker et al. (1994)	3 females (aged 12–15 years) with severe–profound intellectual disability	To increase spontaneous use of manual signed requests	Incomplete/interrupted stimulus presentation and reinforcement of signed requests	With intervention, the number of signed requested increased 138% from baseline levels
Drasgow et al. (1996)	4-year-old girl with severe disability, seizures, and suspected autism	To teach 6 manual signs as requests and 1 natural gesture as a rejecting response	Behavioral indication, time delay, modeling, physical prompting, prompt fading, and reinforcement	With intervention, spontaneous use increased to 100% for 5 of the 6 signs and the natural gesture
Hall and Sundberg (1987)	2 deaf adolescents (aged 16 and 17) with severe intellectual disability	To determine if manual signs taught as tacts would generalize to the manding function	Tact training involved object and signed cues, modeling, and reinforcement. Mand training involved withholding needed objects, tact and imitative prompts, and reinforcement	Manual signs used to tact objects did not occur as mands to request those objects without direct mand training
Sundberg et al. (2000)	2 minimally verbal boys (aged 4 and 5 years) with autism	To teach 6 manual signs as tacts/naming responses	Various types and combinations of prompting (e.g., standard verbal v. intraverbal), modeling, and reinforcement	Correct tacting increased from 0% in baseline to ~50–100% levels with intervention. Intraverbal prompting was more effective than standard prompting
Rudd et al. (2007)	8 students (aged 6–10 years) with moderate-to-severe intellectual disability	To teach productive use of modified signs to express different meaning (e.g., modifying the sign BALL to represent either a big or small ball)	Prompt hierarchy (modeling, imitative and physical), verbal questioning, praise for attending, and reinforcement at end of session	Across children, the percentages of trials with correct use of modified signs increased from the pre-test (~ 6–47%) to the post-test (~18–85)

(continued)

Table 5.1 (continued)

Study	Participants	Intervention goal(s)	Intervention procedures	Outcomes
Scattone and Billhofer (2008)	8-year-old nonverbal boy with autism	To teach 9 manual signs as either mands (4 signs) or tacts (5 signs) and as intraverbal responses (5 of the 9 signs)	Offering/showing object, verbal cuing (e.g., *what do you want?*), modeling, modeling with verbal prompt (e.g., *sign shoe.*), physical prompting, and reinforcement	The child learned to mand in 34–267 trials, to tact in 309–419 trials, and acquired the intraverbal responses in 3–22 trials
Wright et al. (2013)	4 minimally verbal children (aged 23–29 months) with down syndrome	To increase expressive communication/ manual sign use	Simultaneous modeling of signs plus speech during play-based sessions using EMT/ JASPER teaching strategies (see Chap. 3)	Intervention was associated with acquisition of 10–21 manual signs and varied use of 3–9 new spoken words
Meuris et al. (2015)	15 adults (aged 34–74 years) with moderate-to-severe intellectual disability	To teach productive and functional use of 100 signs	Staff were trained to introduce two signs per week using modeling, practice, and verbal and video feedback. Photographs of target signs were posted as reminders	Participants produced significantly more and different signs at post-intervention versus pre-intervention
Frizelle et al. (2023)	36 children (aged 18–61 months) with down syndrome	Examine use of key word signing across book reading conditions with and without key word sign prompts	Key word sign prompts were embedded into a parent–child shared book reading activity	Significantly more signs were attempted when parents embedded key word sign prompts into the shared book reading activity

Note: Studies are listed in alphabetical order by author/author group and then in chronological order by year of publication

while simultaneously speaking the name of the offered item. The child received reinforcement for producing the correct sign (i.e., praise and a portion of the item to eat or drink). If the child did not produce the correct sign, the therapist physically prompted the response while simultaneously saying the object's name.

These procedures were effective in teaching the targeted signs, but a fair amount of training was required for the children to achieve mastery, defined as 10 successive correct responses. Specifically, the four children respectively required 948, 2445, 7279, and 7669 training trials to achieve mastery of the five signs. After training, the children maintained consistently high levels of correct signing and also generalized their use of these signs to other adults. Overall, Carr et al. (1978) demonstrated an effective approach for teaching functional and generalized use of manual signs to nonverbal autistic children. Interestingly, the children's signing was primarily controlled by the visual presentation of each item rather than by the simultaneously presented spoken word. This suggests that the training regime had established the required visual discriminations (e.g., see a cookie and then sign COOKIE), but not the corresponding auditory discriminations (e.g., hear the spoken word *cookie* and then sign COOKIE). Thus, the children in this study did not seem to have benefitted from the simultaneous communication component of the intervention.

However, in a later narrative review of studies employing a simultaneous or total communication approach (i.e., combined use of speech plus manual signing), Goldstein (2002) concluded that "Total communication appears to be a viable treatment strategy for teaching receptive and expressive vocabulary to individuals with autism" (p. 385). Often, total communication is mainly directed toward speech development, rather than establishing manual signing as the person's primary communication strategy (Pattison & Robertson, 2016). Such a focus would seem most applicable for individuals with some propensity to imitate speech, rather than for people who are completely nonverbal.

Following on from their initial 1978 study, Carr and colleagues (Carr et al., 1987; Carr & Kologinsky, 1983) demonstrated that children with autism could learn to produce manual signs under additional antecedent conditions. Carr and Kologinsky, for example, taught six autistic children to make spontaneous manual signed requests when an adult approached. The teaching procedures included physically prompting the children to imitate a signed request and then gradually fading the use of physical prompts. With training, the signed requests came to be used without the adult having to offer preferred objects, as was done in the previous Carr et al. (1978) study. The six children in this 1983 study also learned to produce manual signs without needing a verbal prompt, that is, without the trainer telling the child to make a particular sign. Instead, the six children's signed requests appeared to be more spontaneous in that signing came to be controlled by the mere presence of the adult listener. The children's signing also appeared to function as requests for preferred items as their signing was maintained by the resulting access to the requested items.

Subsequently, in 1987, Carr et al. taught four autistic boys to use manual sign combinations for descriptive purposes, specifically to produce action-object phrases (e.g., MOVE CHAIR and MOVE BALL). Again, a structured intervention approach involving response prompting, prompt fading, and differential reinforcement was shown to be effective for teaching these descriptive sign combinations. Generalized performances (i.e., use of action-object sign combinations that had not been directly taught) emerged during training, although this required a fair amount of instruction, specifically from 1208 to 11,155 training trials.

Studies Involving Adults with Aphasia

The work of Carr and colleagues (Carr et al., 1978, 1987; Carr & Kologinsky, 1983) inspired a research duo, led by Carl Coelho, to explore the use of manual signing with aphasic patients (Coelho, 1987; Coelho & Duffy, 1985, 1986, 1987). In their initial publication, Coelho and Duffy (1985) described outcomes from a sign language training program for a 61-year-old male with nonfluent aphasia secondary to having had a stroke 18 months earlier. His speech was limited to one-word and two-word utterances that were mainly off topic and rote and including some profanity. Signs representing nouns, verbs, and adjectives were taught using a three-step protocol: Imitation, Recognition, and Production. First, the man was taught to imitate a modeled sign. During this step, a picture representing the concept (noun, verb, or adjective) being signed was also present. In the second (Recognition) step, the man had to select the correct picture of the signed concept from an array of four options. Finally, in the Production task, the man had to produce the correct sign when shown the corresponding picture of that concept. A sign was considered to have been acquired when the man produced the correct response in the final Production task. With this training, the man acquired 73 of the 90 targeted signs. However, subsequent tests and observations indicated that the man rarely used the acquired signs spontaneously (i.e., without being shown the corresponding picture) or functionally (e.g., to express a want or need). Similar outcomes were reported in another case study involving a 21-year-old female with severe aphasia and oral–verbal apraxia (Coelho, 1987).

In a larger study, Coelho and Duffy (1986) applied the same Imitation–Recognition–Production training protocol to teach 37 different manual signs to 12 adults with aphasia. The selected target signs varied in terms of iconicity, motoric complexity, and linguistic function (noun, verb, or adjective). The results indicated that signs rated medium to high on the iconicity scale were more readily acquired than signs rated lower on iconicity. Similarly, better acquisition rates were found for motorically less complex signs and for signs representing verbs. In a subsequent analysis of the data, Coelho and Duffy (1987) found that the severity of aphasia influenced sign acquisition. Specifically, acquisition rates were lower for individuals with more severe degrees of aphasia. And, for individuals with the most severe degree of aphasia, "the ability to acquire sign production [was] negligible" (p. 341).

Studies Involving People with Severe and Profound Intellectual Disability

Duker and colleagues (Duker et al., 1991, 1993, 1994; Duker & Michielsen, 1983; Duker & van Lent, 1991; Seys et al., 1990) pursued a significant program of applied-experimental research aimed at developing new and more effective interventions for teaching manual signing to people with severe and profound intellectual disability.

Duker and Michielsen (1983), for example, evaluated a protocol for promoting the initial acquisition of manual signs. In that study, two children and one adolescent with severe intellectual disability received training on three or four manual signs (e.g., MUSIC, DRINK, and DRAW). Instruction began on one sign and once that sign had been acquired, the next sign was taught and so on until all three or four signs had been taught. At the beginning of instruction, the trainer initiated each teaching opportunity by verbalizing the name of the target sign while simultaneously presenting visual cues. Visual cues consisted of showing the object or a picture of the object and modeling the corresponding manual sign. If trainees produced the correct manual sign within 5 s, they received praise and a bite of food or sip of a drink. If the trainee did not produce the correct manual sign, then increasing amounts of physical assistance were delivered until a correct response occurred. When the trainee had made three consecutive correct responses without physical prompting, then the initial modeling cue was removed. Similarly, when correct responding occurred without either physical or model prompts, then the object cue was eliminated. By the end of this intervention, the trainees were correctly producing manual signs when given the verbal cue alone. Achieving this level of performance required from 5–28 sessions or about 2.5–14 hrs of intervention. The signs so acquired in this study also generalized to new settings and people. Similar results were reported in a second study with four additional participants (Duker & Morsink, 1984).

In subsequent studies, Duker and colleagues evaluated procedures for further developing and enhancing participants' use of manual signing. Specifically, Duker and colleagues successfully taught people with severe to profound intellectual disability to (a) make spontaneous requests for preferred and needed stimuli (Duker et al., 1994), (b) increase the variety of manual signs used (Duker & van Lent, 1991), and (c) reject items that did not match their prior signed requests (Duker et al., 1994).

In another important study, Duker et al. (1991) examined the relation between manual signing and problem behavior. The results of this study showed that increasing participants' use of manual signed requests led to a 40% reduction in their self-injurious behavior, a finding that is consistent with the wider literature on functional communication training (see Chap. 3). Such results suggest that early introduction of an alternative communication strategy might be one way to prevent the emergence of self-injury and other forms of problem behavior that are prevalent in this population (Esteves et al., 2021).

Overall the data produced by Duker and colleagues (Duker et al., 1991, 1993, 1994; Duker & Michielsen, 1983; Duker & van Lent, 1991; Seys et al., 1990) has helped to more firmly establish manual signing as a viable communication strategy for nonverbal people with severe to profound intellectual disability. This team's research has been particularly influential in demonstrating that manual signing could be taught in ways that can promote more varied, functional, spontaneous, discriminated, and generalized use of newly acquired manual signs. This program of research has also more firmly established the utility of behavior-analytic/-systematic instructional procedures (e.g., reinforcement and various response prompting, prompt fading, and motivation-boosting strategies) for teaching manual signing to nonverbal people with severe to profound intellectual disability.

Studies Adopting Curriculum Based on Skinner's Analysis of Verbal Behavior

Sundberg and colleagues initiated a significant program of research that integrated behavior-analytic instructional procedures with curricular content based on Skinner's (1957) analysis of verbal behavior (Hall & Sundberg, 1987; Sundberg, 1980; Sundberg et al., 2000; Sundberg & Michael, 2001; Sundberg & Partington, 1998). Skinner's analysis of verbal behavior included a taxonomy of communicative functions, which are now often targeted in contemporary *Applied Verbal Behavior* approaches (LeBlanc et al., 2006; Shillingsburg et al., 2022). Examples of the four main communicative functions often targeted in such communication interventions are the mand, tact, intraverbal, and echoic relations. Table 5.2 provides examples of antecedent conditions and consequences relevant to each of these four main communicative functions.

Table 5.2 Examples of mands, tacts, intraverbals, and echoics

Functions	Antecedent	Response	Reinforcement
Mand	Student needs a spoon to eat his soup Child is thirsty from exercising on a hot day Preschooler needs help tying his shoes	Signs SPOON Signs WATER Signs HELP	Receives the requested spoon from the teacher Receives a glass of water from parent Teacher helps the child tie his shoes
Tact	Child see a dog in the park Child hears front door open Child smells burning toast	Signs DOG Signs MOM + HOME Signs TOAST + BURN	Parent says, *Yes that is a dog. You're smart* Father says *Thanks for letting me know* Mother says *Oh no* and removes toast
Intraverbal	Friend asks *What day can you play tennis?* Peers start singing *Mary had a little* Child asked to name a type of bird	Girl signs MONDAY Child signs LAMB CHILD signs CROW	Friend says *Ok. Good. I will meet you then* Peers smile and nod and continue the song Teacher says *Yes. Crows are a type of bird*
Echoic	A friend says and signs HELLO Teacher signs READY? Teacher models the sign for TREE	Child signs HELLO Child signs READY Child signs TREE	Friend replies *Nice to see you* Teachers replies *Good to hear you are ready* Teacher says *Yes, that's right. You signed tree*

The potential value of combining behavior-analytic instructional tactics with Skinner's (1957) taxonomy of communication behavior was demonstrated in Sundberg's dissertation research (Sundberg, 1980). In this work, Sundberg showed that children with speech and language impairments associated with autism, cerebral palsy, and other developmental disabilities could be taught both expressive and receptive use of manual signing in ways that would enable them to accomplish the range of communicative functions outlined in Table 5.2. To teach expressive signing, for example, one study (Sundberg, 1980, Experiment 3a, pp. 50–55) had the therapist present an object and ask *What is this?* Correct responses were reinforced by providing the object (i.e., correct responses were reinforced as mands). Incorrect responses, in contrast, were followed by a verbal reprimand, verbal instruction, and an imitative prompt. Specifically, the therapist said *no* and modeled the correct sign while instructing the child to *Do this*. If the instruction and imitative prompt did not recruit a correct response, then the correct sign was prompted using varying levels of physical/hand-over-hand guidance.

To teach receptive signing, in contrast, the therapist placed three objects in front of the child and gave the instruction *Touch the [signed object label]*. This receptive language training task could be conceptualized as a type of mand compliance, That is, the child was taught to respond or comply with the therapist's mand/request to *Touch the [signed object label]*. Again, correct responses were reinforced, whereas incorrect responses were subject to a correction procedure, which involved pointing to the correct object, repeating the model of the correct sign, and physical prompting the child to make the correct response, if necessary.

Similar instructional procedures have been successfully used in teaching other types of mands, as well as tacts, intraverbals, and echoic functions. Scattone and Billhofer (2008), for example, reported success in teaching an 8-year-old autistic child to produce manually signed mands, tacts, and intraverbals using the instructional procedures described by Sundberg and Partington (1998). For mand training, the trainer placed a preferred object in view, but out of reach. Preferred objects were cake, gummy worms, a necklace, peanut butter, and a feather. Once the item has been placed, the teacher pointed to the item and asked *What do you want?* In addition, the teacher modeled the correct sign (e.g., CAKE) while also saying the name of the object, that is, the teacher employed a simultaneous modeling approach. Correct responses were reinforced by access to the preferred item. Lack of responding or incorrect responses resulted in the use of a physical prompt. Tact training involved placing one of four objects in front of the child (i.e., hat, shoe, book, or ball) and asking What is this? Correct signed responses resulted in praise and an edible reinforcer. Lack of responding or incorrect signed responses resulted in modeling and physical prompting. Intraverbals included four signs that were also targeted as mands (i.e., PEANUT BUTTER, GUMMY WORM, NECKLACE, and CAKE)) and one sign that was also taught as a tact (i.e., SHOE). Intraverbals were taught by verbally instructing the child to make a particular sign (e.g., *Sign shoe.*). Correct responses were reinforced with praise and an edible. Incorrect responses resulted in modeling and physical prompting. Using these procedures, the child achieved mastery (i.e., unprompted use of the sign on the first opportunity for three consecutive days) of the targeted mands, tacts, and intraverbals in from 3 to 419 trials. Acquisition of tacts required more training trials on average than mands. Intraverbals were acquired most quickly, which likely stems from the fact that four of the five intraverbal signs were previously acquired as mands. However, there was no evidence of any such carry-over effects from mand to tact training, perhaps due to the lack of any common sign topographies. The child also showed an interesting learning-to-learn effect, but only during the initial mand training. Specifically, trials to criterion tended to decrease as mand training on each subsequent sign was introduced.

One assumption or hypothesis arising from Skinner's (1957) analysis is that the basic relations outlined in Table 5.2 are functionally independent. Thus, teaching a child to use a manual sign as a tact, for example, may not necessarily equip the child to use that same sign as a mand and vice versa. One implication arising from this hypothesis is that there may be a need to directly teach the person to use his or her manual signs for each different function or purpose as suggested by the results of Scattone and Billhofer (2008). In line with this implication, Sundberg and colleagues (Sundberg & Michael, 2001; Sundberg & Partington, 1998) have stressed the importance of implementing functionally comprehensive interventions that incorporate mand, tact, intraverbal, and echoic training, rather than an approach aimed at building vocabulary per se.

There is some evidence to support the claim for functional independence of the different communication functions described by Skinner (1957). In a study, involving typically developing children, Lamarre and Holland (1985) showed that responses acquired as requests (i.e., mands) for toy parts were rarely produced when the child was asked to name (i.e., tact) that same toy part and vice versa.

Hall and Sundberg (1987) (see Table 5.1) reported a similar result to that of Lamarre and Holland (1985) in a study involving two profoundly deaf students with severe intellectual disability. The children were first taught to name (i.e., tact) several common objects using manual signs (e.g., CUP, MONEY, and PEN). Once the targeted signs were acquired as tacts, conditions were arranged in which the children needed to request (i.e., mand) these same objects in order to continue a preferred activity. For example, to continue a coloring activity the child had to request a pen and to continue making a cup of instant coffee the child had to request a cup. It is important to note that the topographies of the manual signs being taught were identical for both the tact and mand tasks. In addition, the children knew the objects that they needed for completing their preferred activities. Therefore, any absence of manding after tact acquisition would not have stemmed from simply not knowing that they needed the pen and cup to engage in the coloring and coffee-making activities. The results showed that manual signs learned as tacts did not occur as mands without further and direct mand training.

Studies Evaluating Key Word Signing

Key word signing represents another significant development in the provision of communication intervention for people with severe disabilities (Frizelle et al., 2023; Meuris et al., 2014, 2015). A good example of how the key word signing approach has been implemented in a residential setting for adults with intellectual disability was provided by Meuris et al. (2015). This study involved training 15 support staff to use two new key word signs each week. Staff learned the key word signs and were also taught how to embed the use of these signs into their daily interactions with 15 adults with intellectual disability who were residents of the facility. Pre-post comparisons showed that manual sign usage increased among both the staff and the 15 adults with intellectual disability at a 12-month follow-up. Indeed, the authors reported that all but one of the adults learned to use key word signs in their spontaneous communicative interactions. The results are encouraging as they suggest that spontaneous use of key word signs by adults with intellectual disability can be increased when staff incorporate key word signing into daily interactions.

Another good example of embedding key word signing into natural interactions was published by Frizelle et al. (2023). These authors had parents incorporate key word signing when engaged with their child in a shared book-reading interaction. The participants were 36 children with Down syndrome (aged 18–36 months) and their mothers. Parents engaged the children in a shared book reading activity under two conditions. In one condition, the mothers used a number of key word signs as prompts to engage the child in the shared book reading activity. In the other condition, the mothers did not embed any key word sign prompts. The results showed differences in children's sign usage across conditions with more sign usage and signing attempts during the key word signing condition. The children also showed increased level of attention and initiation during the key word signing condition. Interestingly, the mothers also used more speech in the key word signing condition, although the mean length of their utterances decreased, suggesting parents were simplifying their language usage. These data suggest there is potential value to children with language delays when parents incorporate key word signs into common social interactions, such as a shared book reading activity. The authors of this study further suggested that "embedding KWS in shared book reading is likely to facilitate increased language abilities" (p. 1029). The approach evaluated by Frizelle et al. would seem to represent a reasonable and naturalistic approach for children with delayed speech and language development, such as is the case for children with Down syndrome.

In summary, over the past five decades, a number of high-quality studies have explored strategies for enhancing the use of manual signing as a communication option for nonverbal and minimally verbal people with severe disabilities. Studies of the type summarized in Table 5.1 have collectively demonstrated effective instructional tactics for promoting initial acquisition, as well as generalization and spontaneous/functional use of manual signs and sign combinations by people with severe disabilities. Populations that have been successfully taught to use manual signs and key word signing include nonverbal children and adolescents with autism, children, adolescents, and adults with severe to profound intellectual disability, as well as deaf individuals with severe intellectual disabilities, and people with cerebral palsy, aphasia, and/or traumatic brain injury. Children who exhibit delayed speech and language development, such as children with Down syndrome, can also benefit from interventions that incorporate the use of key word/manual signs as prompts.

Indications for Teaching Manual Signs

Manual signing has several potential advantages and indications for use as a communication strategy for nonverbal and minimally verbal people with severe disabilities. Manual signing may be easier to teach than trying to establish speech because signs can be physically prompted if necessary (Sundberg & Partington, 1998), whereas prompting speech generally requires the person to already have some imitative speech ability. Another potential advantage is portability in the sense manual signing does not require any external materials (Nam et al., 2018). Nam et al. also pointed out that manual signing generally represents a quicker means of message transmission than strategies requiring an external device, such as when the person is required to select symbols from a communication board or tap icons on a speech-generating device.

Another potential advantage is the vast research literature on teaching manual signing to nonverbal and minimally verbal people with severe disabilities. Now spanning over five decades, this literature has resulted in numerous empirically validated instructional procedures. Indeed, research-based procedures can be found that have successfully enabled nonverbal and minimally verbal people with severe disabilities to acquire functional, spontaneous, discriminated, and generalized use of manual signs and to use manual signs to express various important communication functions, as well as participate in meaningful social communicative interactions. Interventions involving the combined use of manual signing and speech (i.e., simultaneous or total communication strategies) might also facilitate natural speech production in some individuals (Goldstein, 2002).

Efforts to establish manual signing may be indicated for individuals who present with delayed or minimal speech and language development. For these individuals, manual signing may represent an important compensatory form of communication as manual signing interventions can be geared toward augmenting the person's limited speech and language. On the other hand, when speech has not developed at all or is so severely impaired that the person is essentially nonverbal, then manual signing may come to represent the person's long-term and primary mode of communication.

Contraindications for Manual Signing

Manual signing is generally contraindicated when physical impairment restricts the person's ability to produce well-articulated signs. Similarly, intervention to teach manual signing might be questioned in cases where learning ability appears to be so significantly impaired that acquisition seems unlikely as was suggested by Coelho and Duffy's (1987) results with severely aphasic patients. However, in such cases it may still be possible to establish a least some simplified manual signs that listeners could learn to recognize and interpret. Bonvillian et al. (2020), for example, described a simplified system of manual signing intended for people with severe forms of aphasia, autism, intellectual disability, and/or cerebral palsy who had difficulty in learning spoken language and/or difficulty in learning a formal sign language. Simplifications included developing motorically uncomplicated and highly iconic (i.e., easily guessable) signs.

The extent to which manual signing would provide an effective communication strategy might also be questioned when the person's communication partners do not know signs. As noted by Nam et al. (2018), "the primary disadvantage [of manual signing] is that communication partners must learn and use manual signs" (p. 10). However, this potential disadvantage can be overcome by upskilling communication partners. For example, by teaching communication partners what the person's signs mean and how to respond to these in ways that would function as effective types of reinforcement.

Along these lines, some research has demonstrated effective procedures for developing listener competencies with respect to recognizing and interpreting manually signed communications emitted by nonverbal persons with severe disabilities. Fitzgerald et al. (1984), for example, successfully taught 34 manual signs to institutional staff involved in the care and habilitation of people with developmental disabilities. Staff were trained using verbal and written instructions, modeling, practice, and feedback. This approach was effective in developing the staff's manual signing skills. Similarly, Seys et al. (1990) used verbal instruction, visual reminders, and feedback in teaching 17 staff how to create opportunities as well as prompt and reinforce manual sign usage among 9 residents in a residential facility for people with intellectual disability. The results showed that staff learned to create opportunities, prompt, and reinforce manual sign use, which in turn lead to increased use of manual signs by the residents.

A different approach to solving the listener-competence issue was described in a unique study by Reichle and Ward (1985). In this study, a 13-year-old boy with intellectual disability first learned to use both manual signs and an aided communication device. Subsequently, the boy was successfully taught to use manual signs when interacting with communication partners who knew signing, but to instead use his aided device with listeners who were not signers. Given that the level of sign language competence is likely to vary within and across cohorts of listeners, there would seem to be considerable value in teaching manual sign users to make use of a back-up communication strategy for situations where knowledge of manual signs among potential communication partners is limited.

Implementation Considerations

For some individuals with severe disabilities, the acquisition of even a relatively small number of manual signs may require many hours of intensive instruction. Interventionists should therefore consider factors that may facilitate the ease and speed of learning. A number of factors are important to consider when designing an intervention to teach, increase, and/or enhance manual signing in people with severe disabilities. The data analyses conducted by Coelho and Duffy (1986, 1987), for example, revealed that iconicity, motoric complexity, linguistic function, and severity of the person's disability influenced the ease of acquisition. Other researchers have also highlighted the importance of considering factors such as sign iconicity and concreteness when selecting an initial vocabulary of manual signs to target for instruction (Luftig & Lloyd, 1981; Meuris et al., 2014).

In addition to factors such as sign iconicity and motoric complexity, the pragmatic function of the sign and its significance to the individual should also be considered. Reichle and colleagues (Reichle et al., 1991; Simacek et al., 2018), for example, have argued for targeting vocabulary (e.g., specific manual signs) that reflect a person's preferred objects and/or activities. Reichle et al. provided rationale for why requesting may represent an appropriate initial communication function to teach. Part of the rationale is that teaching mands for requesting preferred objects will enable the person to express wants and needs and exert some control over reinforcement (Reichle et al., 1991). Thus, even when a sign is motorically complex and opaque it may be acquired if it produces consequences that are highly reinforcing for the individual.

The need to consider motivation is increasingly recognized as a critical factor in communication intervention. Interventions based on Skinner's (1957) analysis of verbal behavior, for example, devote considerable attention to creating the need for communication and capturing the motivational interests of the person (LeBlanc et al., 2006; Shillingsburg et al., 2022; Sundberg & Partington, 1998). It is important to consider that lack of acquisition may indicate reinforcement and motivational problems, rather than reflecting some inherent characteristic of the learner or the signs being taught. For example, some people with severe disabilities may not be motivated by the purely social nature of many communicative interactions. In such cases, the person may respond better when an additional contrived reinforcer (praise plus an unrelated tangible reinforcer) is initially included when teaching manual signs.

The lack of spontaneity observed by Coelho and Duffy (1985) has been frequently reported in the literature on teaching communication skills to people with severe disabilities (Duffy & Healy, 2011; Halle, 1987; Sigafoos, 2021). In the specific case reported by Coelho and Duffy, the lack of spontaneity suggests that while the training protocol had taught the man to correctly name pictures, it did not teach him to use these same manual signs for other communicative purposes, such as for requesting, responding to questions, or initiating a conversation. The lack of spontaneity in this case is consistent with data showing that naming a picture and making a request, for example, are distinct communication functions that often have to be separately taught, even when the response forms used to name and request are identical (Hall & Sundberg, 1987; Lamarre & Holland, 1985). The man's lack of spontaneity is also consistent with the conceptualization of spontaneity as a function of the stimuli that come to control, or set the occasion for, the response during training (Halle, 1987). Spontaneity is predicted to be more limited when training uses a narrow and precisely controlled set of instructional prompts rather than when training incorporates a wider variety of natural cues and prompts and when intervention is incorporated into natural routines and everyday communicative interactions. The possibility of narrow stimulus control is one reason why researchers have become increasingly interested in evaluating the effects of more naturalistic interventions in which key stakeholders (e.g., parents, teachers, and staff) incorporate manual signing and sign training into everyday routines (Wright et al., 2013).

Summary and Conclusion

Manual signing can be a viable and effective communication strategy for people with severe disabilities. Systematic instruction based on principles of applied behavior analysis has considerable empirical support for promoting the acquisition of manual signing in nonverbal and minimally verbal people with severe disabilities. These types of instructional procedures can also be used to establish functional, spontaneous, discriminated, and generalized use of manual signing.

Manual signing is indicated as a primary mode of communication for the nonverbal or minimally verbal individuals who are unlikely to develop sufficient speech to meet their everyday communication needs. Signing may also be indicated to augment speech and language difficulties. Simultaneous use of sign and speech may help advance speech and language development. Manual signing can also be taught as part of a larger multimodal augmentative and alternative communication system (Reichle & Ward, 1985). Contraindications include use with people who lack sufficient motor control to produce intelligible signs and situations where listeners do not understand sign language, although such constraints might be overcome by targeting simplified signs and developing the signing skills of communication partners. Intervention outcomes may improve when interventionists consider the range of factors that are known to facilitate sign learning, such as iconicity, motoric complexity, linguistic function, and motivational factors. Acquisition often requires the provision of numerous learning opportunities. Functional and spontaneous use of newly acquired signs—as well as generalization and discriminated use—are aspects of performance that may often have to be deliberately programmed or directly taught.

References

Beukelman, D. R., & Light, J. C. (2020). *Augmentative and alternative communication: Supporting children and adults with complex communication needs* (5th ed.). Paul H. Brookes Publishing Co.

Bonvillian, J. D., Kissane Lee, N., Dooley, T. T., & Loncke, F. T. (2020). *Simplified signs: A manual sign-communication system for special populations* (Vol. 1). Open Book Publishers. https://doi.org/10.11647/OBP.0205

Carr, E. G. (1979). Teaching autistic children to use sign language: Some research issues. *Journal of Autism and Developmental Disorders, 9*(4), 345–359. https://doi.org/10.1007/BF01531444

Carr, E. G., & Kologinsky, E. (1983). Acquisition of sign language by autistic children II: Spontaneity and generalization effects. *Journal of Applied Behavior Analysis, 16*(3), 297–314. https://doi.org/10.1901/jaba.1983.16-297

Carr, E. G., Binkoff, J. A., Kologinsky, E., & Eddy, M. (1978). Acquisition of sign language by autistic children I: Expressive labelling. *Journal of Applied Behavior Analysis, 11*(4), 489–501. https://doi.org/10.1901/jaba.1978.11-489

Carr, E. G., Kologinsky, E., & Leff-Simon, S. (1987). Acquisition of sign language by autistic children III: Generalized descriptive phrases. *Journal of Autism and Developmental Disorders, 17*(2), 217–229. https://doi.org/10.1007/BF01495057

Coelho, C. A. (1987). Sign acquisition and use following traumatic brain injury: Case report. *Archives of Physical Medicine and Rehabilitation, 68*, 229–231.

Coelho, C. A., & Duffy, R. J. (1985). Communicative use of signs in aphasia: Is acquisition enough? *Clinical Aphasiology, 15*, 222–229.

Coelho, C. A., & Duffy, R. J. (1986). Effects of iconicity, motoric complexity, and linguistic function on sign acquisition in severe aphasia. *Perceptual and Motor Skills, 63*(2), 519–530. https://doi.org/10.2466/pms.1986.63.2.519

Coelho, C. A., & Duffy, R. J. (1987). The relationship of the acquisition of manual signs to severity of aphasia: A training study. *Brain and Language, 31*(2), 328–345. https://doi.org/10.1016/0093-934x(87)90078-2

Crowe, B., Machalicek, W., Wei, Q., Drew, C., & Ganz, J. (2022). Augmentative and alternative communication for children with intellectual and developmental disability: A mega-review of the literature. *Journal of Developmental Physical Disabilities, 34*(1), 1–42. https://doi.org/10.1007/s10882-021-09790-0

Deuchar, M. (2013). *British sign language*. Routledge. https://doi.org/10.4324/9781315005089

Drasgow, E., Halle, J. W., Ostrosky, M. M., & Harbers, H. M. (1996). Using behavioral indication and functional communication training to establish an initial sign repertoire with a young child with severe disabilities. *Topics in Early Childhood Special Education, 16*(4), 500–521. https://doi.org/10.1177/027112149601600408

Duffy, C., & Healy, O. (2011). Spontaneous communication in autism spectrum disorder: A review of topographies and interventions. *Research in Autism Spectrum Disorders, 5*(3), 977–983. https://doi.org/10.1016/j.rasd.2010.12.005

Duker, P. C., & Michielsen, H. M. (1983). Cross-setting generalization of manual signs to verbal instructions with severely retarded children. *Applied Research in Mental Retardation, 4*(1), 29–40. https://doi.org/10.1016/S0270-3092(83)80016-2

Duker, P. C., & Morsink, H. (1984). Acquisition and cross-setting generalization of manual signs with severely retarded individuals. *Journal of Applied Behavior Analysis, 17*(1), 93–103. https://doi.org/10.1901/jaba.1984.17-93

Duker, P. C., & van Lent, C. (1991). Inducing variability in communicative gestures used by severely retarded individuals. *Journal of Applied Behavior Analysis, 24*(2), 379–386. https://doi.org/10.1901/jaba.1991.24-379

Duker, P. C., Jol, K., & Palmen, A. (1991). The collateral decrease of self-injurious behavior with teaching communicative gestures to individuals who are mentally retarded. *Behavioral Residential Treatment, 6*(3), 183–196. https://doi.org/10.1002/bin.2360060304

Duker, P. C., Dortmans, A., & Lodder, E. (1993). Establishing the manding function of communicative gestures with individuals with severe/profound mental retardation. *Research in Developmental Disabilities, 14*(1), 39–49. https://doi.org/10.1016/0891-4222(93)90004-4

Duker, P. C., Kraaykamp, M., & Visser, E. (1994). A stimulus control procedure to increase requesting with individuals who are severely/profoundly intellectually disabled. *Journal of Intellectual Disability Research, 38*(2), 177–186. https://doi.org/10.1111/j.1365-2788.1994.tb00372.x

Esteves, J., Perry, A., Spiegel, R., & Weiss, J. A. (2021). Occurrence and predictors of challenging behavior in youth with intellectual disability with or without autism. *Journal of Mental Health Research in Intellectual Disability, 14*(2), 189–201. https://doi.org/10.1080/19315864.2021.1874577

Fitzgerald, J. R., Reid, D. H., Schepis, M. M., Faw, G. D., Welty, P. A., & Pyfer, L. M. (1984). A rapid training procedure for teaching manual sign language skills to multidisciplinary institutional staff. *Applied Research in Mental Retardation, 5*(4), 451–469. https://doi.org/10.1016/s0270-3092(84)80038-7

Frizelle, P., Allenby, R., Hassett, E., Holland, O., Ryan, E., Dahly, D., & O'Toole, C. (2023). Embedding key word sign prompts in a shared book reading activity: The impact on communication between children with down syndrome and their parents. *International Journal of Language & Communication Disorders, 58*(4), 1029–1045. https://doi.org/10.1111/1460-6084-12842

Fuller, D. R., & Pampoulou, E. (2022). Opinion: Revisiting the means to select and transmit of the AAC model. *Journal of Enabling Technologies, 16*(1), 321–339. https://doi.org/10.1108/JET-09-2021-0044

Ganz, J. B. (2014). *Aided augmentative communication for individuals with autism spectrum disorders*. Springer. https://doi.org/10.1007/978-1-4939-0814-1

Goldstein, H. (2002). Communication intervention for children with autism: A review of treatment efficacy. *Journal of Autism and Developmental Disorders, 32*(5), 373–396. https://doi.org/10.1023/a:1020589821992

Grove, N., & Dockrell, J. (2000). Multisign combinations by children with intellectual impairment: An analysis of language skills. *Journal of Speech, Language, and Hearing Research, 43*(2), 309–323. https://doi.org/10.1044/jslhr.4302.309

Grove, N., & Walker, M. (1990). The Makaton vocabulary: Using manual signs and graphic symbols to develop interpersonal communication. *Augmentative and Alternative Communication, 6*(1), 15–27. https://doi.org/10.1080/07434619012331275284

Hall, G., & Sundberg, M. L. (1987). Teaching mands by manipulating conditioned establishing operations. *Analysis of Verbal Behavior, 5*(1), 41–53. https://doi.org/10.1007/BF03392819

Halle, J. W. (1987). Teaching language in the natural environment: An analysis of spontaneity. *Journal of the Association for Persons with Severe Handicaps, 12*(1), 28–37. https://doi.org/10.1177/154079698701200105

Johnston, T., & Schembri, A. (2007). *Australian sign language (Auslan): An introduction to sign language linguistics*. Cambridge University Press.

Kleinert, H. L., & Gast, D. L. (1981). Teaching a multihandicapped adult manual signs using a constant time delay procedure. *Journal of the Association for the Severely Handicapped, 6*(4), 25–32. https://doi.org/10.1177/154079698200600404

Lamarre, J., & Holland, J. G. (1985). The functional independence of mands and tacts. *Journal of the Experimental Analysis of Behavior, 43*(1), 5–19. https://doi.org/10.1901/jeab.1985.43-5

Leblanc, L. A., Esch, J., Sidener, T. M., & Firth, A. M. (2006). Behavioral language interventions for children with autism: Comparing applied verbal behavior and naturalistic teaching approaches. *The Analysis of Verbal Behavior, 22*(1), 49–60. https://doi.org/10.1007/BF03393026

Luftig, R. L., & Lloyd, L. L. (1981). Manual sign translucency and referential concreteness in the learning of signs. *Sign Language Studies, 30*(1), 49–60. https://doi.org/10.1353/sls.1981.0005

Meuris, K., Maes, B., De Meyer, A., & Zink, I. (2014). Manual signing in adults with intellectual disability: Influence of sign characteristics on functional sign vocabulary.

Journal of Speech, Language, and Hearing Research, 57(3), 990–1010. https://doi.org/10.1044/2014_JSLHR-L-12-0402

Meuris, K., Maes, B., & Zink, I. (2015). Teaching adults with intellectual disability manual signs through their support staff: A key word signing program. *American Journal of Speech-Language Pathology, 24*(3), 545–560. https://doi.org/10.1044/2015_AJSLP-14-0062

Nam, S., Kim, J., & Sparks, S. (2018). An overview of review studies on effectiveness of major AAC systems for individuals with developmental disabilities including autism. *The Journal of Special Education Apprenticeship, 7*(2), 1–14. https://doi.org/10.58729/2167-3454.1071

Pattison, A. E., & Robertson, R. E. (2016). Simultaneous presentation of speech and sign prompts to increase MLU in children with intellectual disability. *Communication Disorders Quarterly, 37*(3), 141–147. https://doi.org/10.1177/1525740115583633

Reichle, J., & Ward, M. (1985). Teaching discriminative use of an encoding electronic communication device and signing exact English to a moderately handicapped child. *Language, Speech, and Hearing Services in Schools, 16*(1), 58–63. https://doi.org/10.1044/0161-1461.1601.58

Reichle, J., York, J., & Sigafoos, J. (1991). *Implementing augmentative and alternative communication: Strategies for learners with severe disabilities*. Paul H. Brookes Publishing Co.

Remington, B., & Clarke, S. (1983). Acquisition of expressive signing by autistic children: An evaluation of the relative effects of simultaneous communication and sign alone training. *Journal of Applied Behavior Analysis, 16*(3), 315–327. https://doi.org/10.1901/jaba.1983.16-315

Rudd, H., Grove, N., & Pring, T. (2007). Teaching productive sign modifications to children with intellectual disabilities. *Augmentative and Alternative Communication, 23*(2), 154–163. https://doi.org/10.1080/07434610601124867

Scattone, D., & Billhofer, B. (2008). Teaching sign language to a nonvocal child with autism. *The Journal of Speech and Language Pathology — Applied Behavior Analysis, 3*(1), 78–85. https://doi.org/10.1037/h0100234

Seys, D., Kersten, H., & Duker, P. C. (1990). Evaluating a ward staff program for increasing spontaneous and varied communicative gesturing with individuals who are mentally retarded. *Behavioral Residential Treatment, 5*(4), 247–257. https://doi.org/10.1002/bin.2360050404

Shillingsburg, M. A., Frampton, S. E., Juban, B., Weddle, S. A., & Silva, M. R. (2022). Implementing an applied verbal behavior model in classrooms. *Behavioral Interventions, 37*(1), 56–78. https://doi.org/10.1002/bin.1807

Sigafoos, J. (2021). Teaching communication skills to people with intellectual and developmental disabilities. In R. Lang & P. Sturmey (Eds.), *Adaptive behavior strategies for individuals with intellectual and developmental disabilities* (pp. 73–102). Springer. https://doi.org/10.1007/978-3-030-66441-1_4

Simacek, J., Reichle, J., Byiers, B. J., Parker-McGowan, Q., Dimian, A. F., & Elmquist, M. (2018). Promoting conditional use of communication skills for learners with complex communication needs: A tutorial. *American Journal of Speech-Language Pathology, 27*(2), 519–535. https://doi.org/10.1044/2017_AJSLP-17-0058

Skinner, B. F. (1957). *Verbal behavior*. Appleton-Century-Crofts.

Stewart, D. A., & Stewart, J. (2021). *Barron's American sign language: A comprehensive guide to ASL 1 and 2*. Simon & Schuster.

Sundberg, M. L. (1980). *Developing a verbal repertoire using sign language and Skinner's analysis of verbal behavior*. Dissertations. 2606. https://scholarworks.wmich.edu/dissertations/2606

Sundberg, M. L., & Michael, J. (2001). The benefits of Skinner's analysis of verbal behavior for children with autism. *Behavior Modification, 25*(5), 698–724. https://doi.org/10.1177/0145445501255003

Sundberg, M. L., & Partington, J. W. (1998). *Teaching language to children with autism and other developmental disabilities*. AVB Press.

Sundberg, M. L., Endicott, K., & Eigenheer, P. (2000). Using intraverbal prompts to establish tacts for children with autism. *The Analysis of Verbal Behavior, 17*, 89–104. https://doi.org/10.1007/BF03392958

Syriopoulou-Delli, C. K., & Eleni, G. (2022). Effectiveness of different types of augmentative and alternative communication (AAC) in improving communication skills and in enhancing the vocabulary of children with ASD: A review. *Review Journal of Autism and Developmental Disorders, 9*(4), 493–506. https://doi.org/10.1007/s40489-021-00269-4

Wright, C. A., Kaiser, A. P., Reikowsky, D. I., & Roberts, M. Y. (2013). Effects of a naturalistic sign intervention on expressive language of toddlers with down syndrome. *Journal of Speech, Language, and Hearing Research, 56*(3), 994–1008. https://doi.org/10.1044/1092-4388(2012/12-0060)

Chapter 6
Use of Tangible Symbols

Introduction

In the field of augmentative and alternative communication, tangible symbols represent a type of aided communication system. Tangible symbol sets typically consist of three-dimensional miniature objects or parts of objects that relate in some way to corresponding real-world referents. Generally, the communicative act associated with use of tangible symbols consists of touching, picking up, handing over, or pointing to the tangible symbols, which is considered functionally equivalent to speaking a word or phrase.

Rowland and Schweigert (2009) listed a number of different types of materials that could serve as the basis for a tangible symbol system, including (a) whole objects, (b) parts of objects, (c) objects associated with an activity, and (d) various textures and shapes. Trief et al. (2009) stated that a tangible symbol set could incorporate objects or partial objects that "share a perceptual relationship" with their corresponding referent and that those referents could be "a person, place, object, activity, or concept" (p. 425). Most of the tangible symbols that have been used in the research literature to date have been purposefully constructed on an individual basis. However, there have been some efforts to develop standardized tangible symbol sets. Trief et al. (2009), for example, developed a set of 55 different tangible symbol-referent combinations (e.g., paint brush-art class, magnet-science class, and timer-break time) based on a survey of teachers, speech-language pathologists, and other educational professionals. This set was intended for use in school settings serving prelinguistic and visually impaired children.

Key features of tangible symbols include the fact that they are (a) permanent, rather than fleeting, (b) capable of being physically manipulated using simple motor

J. Sigafoos et al., *Communication Strategies for People with Severe Disabilities*,
Autism and Child Psychopathology Series,
https://doi.org/10.1007/978-3-031-83807-1_6

acts, such as touch and grasp, for example, and (c) discriminable by shape, size, and/or texture. Researchers have suggested that these features of tangible symbol systems may be beneficial for individuals with significant intellectual impairment because they may place lower cognitive demands on the person's short-term memory (Rowland & Schweigert, 2000; Trief et al., 2009). However, there appears to be relatively little experimental research into the cognitive demands associated with different augmentative and alternative communication strategies (Fried-Oken et al., 2019; Thistle & Wilkinson, 2013). In addition, when considering the use of different communication strategies for nonverbal/minimally verbal people with severe disabilities, the practical benefits, if any, of attempts to assess cognitive load remain unclear. On the other hand, observations of typical language development suggest that tangible objects have a foundational role in "shaping children's first communicative acts" (Guevara & Rodŕiguez, 2023, p. 1). Such observations of early language development would seem to support the use of tangible symbols for individuals with severe disabilities because many such individuals are likely to be functioning at an early or beginning stage of communication development (Reichle et al., 2002).

Fig. 6.1 provides an example of a tangible symbol board that could be used to enable a person to choose among different beverages (i.e., milk, orange juice, and coffee) and foods (i.e., hamburger, sandwich, and pizza). The tangible symbol board shown in Fig. 6.1 consists of small (about 10 × 4 × 4 cm) cardboard cartons and miniature plastic objects (about 2 × 2 × 2 cm) that resemble the corresponding actual real items to a certain degree. Fig. 6.2 provides an example of a tangible symbol board that could be used to enable an adolescent to request participation in different leisure activities (i.e., playing basketball in the school gymnasium, walking the family dog, and going skateboarding at the neighborhood skate park).

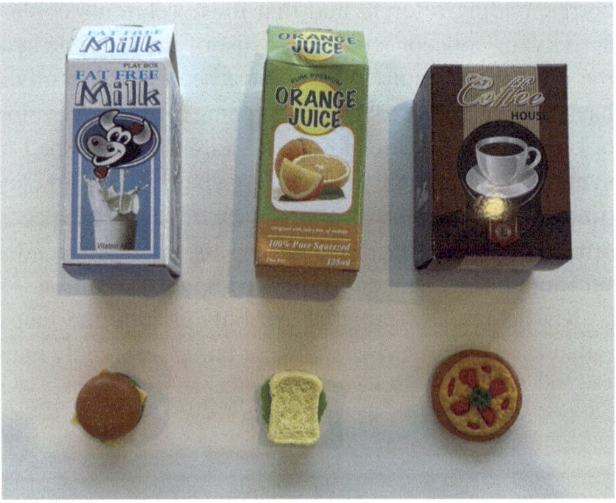

Fig. 6.1 Example of a tangible symbol board for choosing foods and beverages

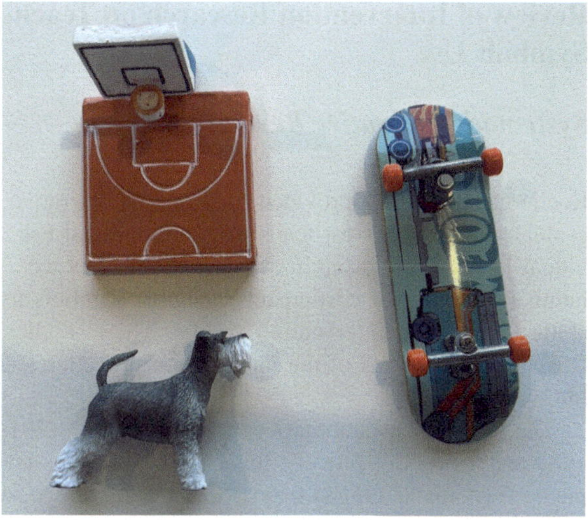

Fig. 6.2 Example of a tangible symbol board for choosing leisure activities

Tangible symbols vary in terms of the extent to which they resemble their corresponding real-world referents. When a tangible symbol closely resembles its real-world referent, it could be considered more transparent or guessable (Schlosser et al., 2012). When considering communicative partners in the exchange, the more transparent the symbol, the more likely its meaning can be readily deciphered. Highly transparent symbols might therefore facilitate communication interactions across multiple partners and contexts. For example, the miniature skateboard in Fig. 6.2 bears a fairly close resemblance to an actual skateboard. Thus, if a child were to pick up that tangible symbol when asked *What do you want to do today?*, the parent would most likely understand that their child was indicating a desire to go skateboarding. In contrast, the meaning of a small square of blanket material to represent naptime or bedtime could be seen as less readily guessable until both the child and his or her communication partners have learned its meaning. Learning the meaning of a tangible symbol may occur as part of the intervention process.

The functional value of the person's tangible symbols is also likely to influence the ease and speed of acquisition. Touching a tangible symbol that represents a highly preferred object may be readily acquired as a requesting response, for example, even if that symbol is not particularly transparent. Indeed, Sevcik et al. (2018) noted that the iconicity or transparency of communication symbols may not necessarily be "a critical factor in learning a symbol-referent relationship" (p. 265). What may be more important is the extent to which appropriate evidence-based instructional strategies are implemented with fidelity. To that end, the next section reviews intervention studies focused on teaching the functional use of tangible symbols to nonverbal and minimally verbal individuals with severe disabilities.

Review of Intervention Research on Teaching Tangible Symbols Use

Systematic-Narrative Review

Roche et al. (2014a) provided a systematic-narrative review of nine studies that evaluated procedures for teaching the functional use of tangible symbols to individuals with severe disabilities. The nine studies were summarized in terms of the number and ages of participants, tangible symbols used, type of communication skills taught, and intervention results. These studies were also summarized by Roche et al. in terms of the intervention procedures and designs used to evaluate intervention effects.

The nine studies summarized by Roche et al. (2014a) were published between 1989 and 2014. Collectively, this cohort of studies involved a total of 129 participants. Participants ranged from 3 to 20 years of age, with most being school-aged students. Most of these 129 participants had a combination of intellectual, physical, and/or sensory impairments. The types of tangible symbols used across the nine studies consisted mainly of three-dimensional objects that related in some way to corresponding real-world referents. For example: (a) real objects (e.g., a plastic spoon to represent having lunch in the school cafeteria), (b) parts of real objects (e.g., a handlebar grip to represent bike riding), (c) miniature figurines of corresponding real objects, such as the symbols shown in Fig. 6.1, and (d) objects that had a similar texture to a real-world counterpart (e.g., a sample of blanket material to represent naptime or bedtime).

All nine studies summarized by Roche et al. (2014a) focused on teaching participants to use tangible symbols to make requests and/or choices. In addition, three of the nine studies also targeted the naming or tact function (Rowland & Schweigert, 1989, 2000; Trief, 2007). One study (Trief et al., 2013) had the relatively ambitious goal of teaching participants to use their tangible symbols for four distinct communicative functions, that is, (a) requesting/choice making, (b) naming, (c) directing the actions of others, and (d) for transitions.

In terms of intervention procedures employed to teach the targeted communication skills, most of the nine studies summarized by Roche et al. (2014a) used multicomponent intervention packages consisting of various combinations of well-established instructional procedures. The specific instructional strategies used were similar to the types of tactics that have proven to be generally effective in teaching prelinguistic responses, natural gestures, and also manual signs to persons with severe disabilities (see Chaps. 3, 4, 5). Specifically, Rowland and Schweigert (1989) created learning opportunities by offering preferred stimuli (objects and activities) and then prompting and reinforcing the child's correct use of tangible symbols. Turnell and Carter (1994) used an intervention package consisting of four components (i.e., expectant look, time delay, modeling, and natural reinforcement). These procedures were successful in teaching an 8-year-old child with severe/multiple disabilities to use tangible symbols to request preferred leisure activities. Rowland

and Schweigert (2000) used a combination of time delay, response prompting, prompt fading, error correction, and differential reinforcement in teaching naming and requesting responses via a tangible symbol board. Trief (2007) implemented an intervention consisting of verbal cueing, response prompting, and error correction to teach the use of tangible symbols for requesting and naming functions. Three studies (Ali et al., 2011; Lund & Troha, 2008; Parker et al., 2010) used a modified version of Bondy and Frost's (1994, 1998; Frost & Bondy, 2002), Picture Exchange Communication System (see Chap. 7), to teach the use of tangible symbols as requesting responses.

In terms of intervention outcomes, data from the nine studies indicated that a slight majority of the 129 participants (i.e., $n = 74$ or 54%) learned to use at least one tangible symbol as a means of communicating. Acquisition of targeted symbols to the 80–100% level was reported in five studies (i.e., Ali et al., 2011; Lund & Troha, 2008; Parker et al., 2010; Roche et al., 2014b; Turnell & Carter, 1994). In these five studies, the acquisition criteria were always achieved within 30 intervention sessions and generally each session in these studies lasted about 10–15 min. It is suggestive to note that these five studies focused on teaching requests and employed well-established instructional procedures (e.g., time delay, response prompting, and natural reinforcement) to do so. Similarly positive results were reported by Rowland and Schweigert (1989). These researchers also applied response prompting and reinforcement in teaching nine participants to make requests/choices and name objects. The participants learned from 16 to 98 symbols over the 10–19-month intervention. Rowland and Schweigert (2000), in contrast, reported more mixed results, but still most ($n = 35$ or 85%) of their 41 participants did learn to make requests with tangible symbols. Trief and colleagues (Trief, 2007; Trief et al., 2013) also reported mixed outcomes. In the first of these two studies, the reported outcomes for a sample of 25 children were that (a) 5 children learned 28 symbols, (b) 10 learned from 1 to 20 symbols, but (c) 10 children did not learn any symbols. In the second study, Trief et al. reported no significant pre-post gains for a sample of 43 participants, although there was some increase in tangible symbol use from the first month to the final month of intervention.

Overall, Roche et al.'s (2014a) review suggested that "tangible symbols appear promising" as a communication strategy (p. 28) for nonverbal children and adolescents with severe and multiple disabilities, including children with significant visual impairment/blindness. Indeed, outcomes appeared particularly strong when intervention focused on teaching the requesting function using well-established systematic instructional tactics, specifically (a) creating discrete requesting opportunities by offering preferred objects, (b) prompting tangible symbol use, (c) gradually fading prompts over successive opportunities, and (d) providing natural reinforcement contingent on the child's use of a tangible symbol (i.e., the child received the preferred item represented by the tangible symbol).

However, these conclusions should be interpreted with caution given the relatively few number of studies included in the Roche et al. (2014a) review. In addition, more than half of the nine studies, which included the vast majority of participants (i.e., $n = 119$ or 92% of the participants), used pre-experimental or quasi-experimental designs to evaluate intervention effects. The use of pre-experimental and quasi-experimental designs reduces the certainty of evidence provided by these studies. Only four studies, including a total of 10 participants, used experimental designs that were capable of ruling out major threats to internal validity and therefore capable of providing convincing evidence of a positive intervention effect. In conclusion, the studies reviewed by Roche et al. provide suggestive evidence to support the use of systematic instructional procedures for teaching children and adolescents with severe/multiple disabilities and significant visual impairment/blindness to make requests using tangible symbols.

More Recent Intervention Studies

Four additional studies on teaching tangible symbol use—which were published after the Roche et al. (2014a) review—are summarized in Tables 6.1 and 6.2. Table 6.1 summarizes these four studies in terms of the number and ages of the participants, tangible symbols used, communication skills targeted for intervention, and intervention outcomes. Table 6.2 provides a summary of the intervention procedures and evaluation/research designs used in each of these four more recent studies.

Cascella (2014) addressed the question of whether a 53-year-old man (Frank) could learn to use a tangible symbol plus a switch device to more directly request a beverage during morning and afternoon breaktimes at an adult day program. Frank was described as having a profound intellectual disability and autism spectrum disorder. He was also classified as legally blind. Communication assessments completed prior to intervention indicated that Frank communicated primarily through direct pre-symbolic means, such as pushing away undesired items and reaching for items he wanted. He did not speak any words nor use gestures or manual signs.

The goal for Frank was to use a two-step tangible symbol sequence to request a drink. This goal was selected because staff noted that during breaktimes Frank would often just stand up, seemingly to indicate that he wanted to get a drink, but he did not indicate this request in any more specific or obviously communicative way. The tangible symbols for Frank consisted of two plastic cups and the goal was to teach him to touch each cup in sequence. Intervention occurred at his morning and afternoon breaks. One symbol, consisting of a plastic cup, was placed within reach. The other symbol, exemplified in Fig. 6.3, consisted of a plastic cup affixed to a switch device. This was located near a refrigerator where the beverages were stored. After an initial baseline (A phase), during which no prompting occurred, the initial errorless training sessions (B phase) involved explaining and modeling use of the tangible symbols. Next, in the subsequent third or C phase of intervention, Frank was prompted to touch the symbols in sequence using a mixture of modeling and physical, gesture, and verbal prompts. After touching the first symbol, Frank would then be guided toward the second symbol located near the refrigerator and prompted to touch that second switch-mounted symbol, which activated the recorded message (*I'd LIKE A DRINK.*). Natural reinforcement (receiving a beverage) was provided

Table 6.1 Summary of four additional intervention studies on teaching tangible symbols to people with severe disabilities

Study	Participants	Tangible symbols	Target skills	Outcomes
Cascella (2014)	A 53-year-old legally blind and nonverbal man with profound intellectual disability and autism	Two clear plastic cups were used as symbols. One cup was mounted on a poster board and the other was affixed to a switch that produced the recorded message *I'd LIKE A DRINK PLEASE*.	The man was taught to hand over or touch the tangible symbols to request a drink.	Before intervention, the man did not independently use the tangible symbols to request a drink during break sessions. During intervention, independent use of the tangible symbols averaged 70% and increased to 80% across the final 10 requesting opportunities.
Ivy et al. (2014)	4 nonverbal boys (aged 5–11 years) with severe visual and cognitive impairment	Cardboard embedded with whole or partial objects representing preferred stimuli.	Picking up the correct tangible symbol and handing it over to the communication partner to request the corresponding preferred item. The response involved four steps: (a) pick up symbol, (b) extending the symbol toward the communication partner, (c) letting go of the symbol after extending it to partner, and (d) moving toward the partner when the partner was distant.	Before intervention, correct use of tangible symbols was 0%. With intervention, all four participants reached mastery (80% correct over 3 successive sessions) on the initial (Phase 1) target skill (i.e., exchanging tangible symbols to request preferred stimuli). Mastery occurred within 7–14 days or 3.5–7 h of instruction. One child also learned to approach a distant partner.

(continued)

Table 6.1 (continued)

Study	Participants	Tangible symbols	Target skills	Outcomes
Ivy et al. (2020)	3 nonverbal/minimally verbal children (aged 4–7 years) with hearing loss and developmental disability syndromes	Tangible objects (5 × 7 cm) resembling the tactual, auditory, and/or visual characteristics of preferred items. For example, a preferred snack was represented by its wrapper.	Picking up the correct tangible symbol and handing it over to the communication partner to request the corresponding preferred item. Responding involved four discrete steps: (a) pick up symbol, (b) extending the symbol toward the communication partner, (c) letting go of the symbol after extending it to partner, and (d) moving toward the partner when the partner was distant.	Before intervention, correct use of tangible symbols was 0%. With intervention, all three children reached mastery (80% correct or better over 3 consecutive sessions) within 2.8–6 h of intervention. The children also learned to activate a speech-generating device to recruit the partner's attention before making a request. Correct responding generalized to a new partner and to a distant partner (3 m away).
Sutter and Demchak (2023)	A nonverbal and deafblind girl (aged 15 years) who also likely had intellectual disability[a]	The girl was taught to make three requests by touching three tangible objects.	Selecting/touching symbols to request corresponding preferred items or activities (e.g., touching a 30 cm mermaid doll to request music from the *Little Mermaid* movie).	Before intervention, correct symbol use ranged from 0–20%. With intervention, the girl reached criterion (80% over 3 sessions) on the first tangible symbol after 24 sessions. On the second symbol, correct use increased from 20 to 80% over the final 8 sessions. On the third symbol, correct use during intervention stabilized at about 20–40% over the final four sessions.

[a]*Note*. The Sutter and Demchak (2023) study included two participants, but only one participant was taught to use tangible symbols

Table 6.2 Summary of the intervention procedures and designs used in the Cascella (2014), Ivy et al. (2014, 2020), and Sutter and Demchak (2023) studies

Study	Intervention procedures	Evaluation design
Cascella (2014)	Errorless learning phase involved verbal instruction and modeling. Subsequent intervention phases involved modeling and physical, gestural, and verbal prompts. Responses produced natural reinforcement.	Pre-experimental: an initial baseline phase without prompting was followed by three intervention phases, in a sequential ABCD design
Ivy et al. (2014)	Modified PECS protocol: Phases 1 and 2.	Experimental: multiple probe design across participants
Ivy et al. (2020).	Modified PECS protocol: Phases 1 and 2.	Experimental: multiple probe design across participant.
Sutter and Demchak (2023)	Verbal cueing, system of least (physical) prompts, stimulus (positioning) prompt, differential social reinforcement, and natural reinforcement.	Experimental: multiple probe design across three tangible symbols

Note. PECS refers to the Picture Exchange Communication System (Bondy & Frost, 1994, 1998; Frost & Bondy, 2002)

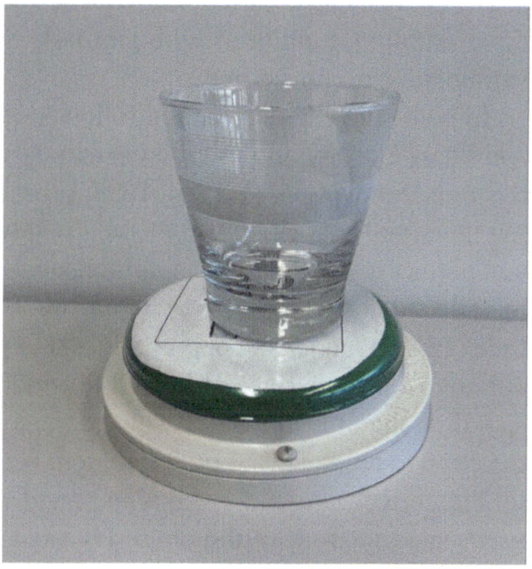

Fig. 6.3 Example of the type of tangible symbol plus switch system described by Cascella (2014)

for correct responses. In the final intervention sessions (D phase), prompting was not used so as to promote more independent and spontaneous use of the two-step tangible symbol sequence (Fig. 6.3).

As summarized in Table 6.1, application of the intervention procedures was associated with Frank rather quickly learning to engage in the two-step tangible symbol sequence without prompting. Specifically, across the 10 initial baseline opportunities, Frank never completed the sequence. His first independent (i.e., unprompted) use of the tangible symbols occurred on the fourth intervention opportunity. With continued intervention, independent use of the tangible symbols increased and eventually occurred during the majority of his requesting opportunities. In total, Frank received 30 intervention opportunities and produced an independent response on 21 (or 70%) of these opportunities.

These results are encouraging given the severity of Frank's intellectual, visual, and communication impairments. Frank gained independence in using a rather unique and innovative two-step tangible symbol sequence that included a speech-generating device. The fact that a clear learning effect was evidenced within relatively few teaching opportunities suggests that the prompting procedures employed were well suited to Frank's situation. Frank's rapid acquisition also suggests that the two plastic cups represented a meaningful and practical type of tangible symbol system for him. Access to beverages as a consequence for using the tangible symbols also appeared to be a powerful reinforcer sufficient to maintain Frank's independent use of the tangible symbols even without prompting, which was the case during the final 10 opportunities.

Two studies by Ivy and colleagues (Ivy et al., 2014, 2020) adapted the Picture Exchange Communication System (Bondy & Frost, 1994, 1998; Frost & Bondy, 2002) for use with tangible symbols. Specifically, Ivy et al. (2014) successfully taught four nonverbal boys with severe vision and cognitive impairments to exchange tangible symbols (e.g., an empty snack package, a plastic cup, and a small rubber ball) to request corresponding reinforcers (e.g., cheese crackers, juice, and a larger rubber ball). In the subsequent study, Ivy et al. (2020) successfully taught three additional children with similarly severe impairments to exchange tangible symbols for preferred items.

In both studies, intervention followed the procedures associated with the Phase 1 and Phase 2 protocols described in manuals for the Picture Exchange Communication System (Bondy & Frost, 1994, 1998; Frost & Bondy, 2002). Phase 1 focuses on teaching the initial exchange, and Phase 2 involves teaching individuals to approach a distant partner to complete the communicative exchange (see Chap. 7). Training occurred in daily structured sessions of about 10–30 min, with each session consisting of multiple (15–50) requesting opportunities. For each requesting opportunity in Phase 1, the communication partner presented a preferred item and showed the child its corresponding tangible symbol. A second person (positioned behind the child) waited for the child to reach for the preferred item before physically prompting the child to pick up the correct tangible symbol and hand it to the first communication partner, who was seated in front of the child. Physical prompting was systematically faded over successive requesting opportunities, whereas errors were followed by increasing the amount of physical assistance provided. Correct symbol exchanges were reinforced by providing access to the corresponding preferred item. Once this initial exchange had been mastered (i.e., 80% correct over three successive sessions), Phase 2 training was implemented. Phase 2 training aimed to teach the children to first approach a distant partner (Ivy et al., 2014) or to first recruit the attention of a distant partner by activating a speech-generating device (Ivy et al., 2020). These Phase 2 skills were taught using prompting, error correction, and reinforcement. Ivy et al. (2020) also included generalization sessions with a new communicative partner.

In both studies, Ivy and colleagues (Ivy et al., 2014, 2020) evaluated intervention effects experimentally using multiple-probe across participants' designs. With intervention, all of the participating children learned to exchange tangible symbols to make requests within 12–17 sessions or in about 3–7 instructional hours. However, only one of the four children in Ivy et al. (2014) learned the Phase 2 skill of approaching a distant partner. In contrast, two of the three children in the Ivy et al. (2020) study learned to use the speech-generating device to first recruit attention and then complete the exchange. For these two children, acquisition of the complete sequence (i.e., recruit attention and then exchange the tangible symbol) occurred within 8–13 sessions or about 2–3 instructional hours. The third child in the Ivy et al. (2020) study also showed gains in the more advanced Phase 2 intervention sessions, but fell just below the preset mastery criterion.

Collectively, the data generated by Ivy and colleagues (Ivy et al., 2014, 2020) further demonstrate the feasibility of adapting the Picture Exchange Communication System (Bondy & Frost, 1994, 1998; Frost & Bondy, 2002) to a tangible symbol system. These results are consistent with the findings reported by Ali et al. (2011), Lund and Troha (2008), and Parker et al. (2010). Ivy et al.'s (2014, 2020) data provide much-needed replication evidence and also help extend the literature given that most of the work with the Picture Exchange Communication System has mainly involved teaching autistic children to exchange two-dimensional picture cards (see Chap. 7). However, some of Ivy et al.'s participants failed to acquire the approach and attention recruitment skills targeted in Phase 2. It is possible that their significant vision impairments may have made it more difficult for these children to discriminate whether the communication partner was present and attending versus distant and/or not attending. In such cases, additional discrimination training procedures may be indicated.

Sutter and Demchak (2023) provided communication intervention to two children, but only one of these children (i.e., Beth) was taught to use tangible symbols. This participant and her intervention details are summarized in Tables 6.1 and 6.2. Specifically, Beth was a nonverbal 15-year-old girl who was described as having multiple impairments including being deafblind. Her tangible symbol set consisted of three-dimensional, brightly colored objects mounted on 20 × 20 cm boards. Her symbols were a pink squishy ball, a *Little Mermaid* doll, and a cup. During intervention, use of these symbols was followed by the trainer naming the object, praising the response (*Ball. Nice asking for the ball.*) as well as giving Beth the corresponding reinforcer (i.e., giving her a larger ball to play with, playing a sample of music from the *Little Mermaid* movie, or giving Beth a cup containing preferred foods or drinks).

Sessions, consisting of 5–10 requesting opportunities, occurred three times per day, with each session focusing on teaching Beth to request one reinforcer by selecting its corresponding tangible symbol. Intervention initially consisted of presenting a verbal cue (*Tell me what you want.*). If Beth did not respond within 5 s, the trainer used a system of least prompts (i.e., touch/tap the back of Beth's hand, give a partial physical prompt, and give a full physical prompt). To counter Beth's initially slow acquisition, additional social reinforcers (i.e., more enthusiastic praise, back rubs, and hugs) were delivered along with the requested stimulus whenever Beth responded to the less intrusive touch prompt. If Beth needed more intrusive assistance (i.e., a partial or full physical prompt), then she received only quiet praise plus access to the requested item. In addition, when teaching the *Little Mermaid* symbol, an additional stimulus prompt was added (i.e., the *Little Mermaid* symbol was placed 5 cm closer to Beth) to make it easier for her to discriminate between the *Little Mermaid* symbol and the pink squishy ball symbol).

The effects of the intervention were evaluated in a multiple-probe across symbols design. In baseline, Beth made a few independent responses in response to the verbal cue *Tell me what you want.* Specifically, she had no independent responses in 29 of the 32 total baseline sessions. For the three baseline sessions where some independent responding did occur (which occurred in only one session for each symbol), the percentage of opportunities with an independent response never exceeded 20. With intervention, Beth showed a gradually accelerating trend in terms of the percentage of opportunities with independent use of the first (ball) symbol. At the end of this first leg of her intervention, Beth had reached the 80% level and maintained at 50–80% during three maintenance sessions. Progress was also seen when intervention was extended to the second (*Little Mermaid*) symbol. By the end of the 21 intervention sessions conducted on that symbol, Beth was independently requesting music by selecting the *Little Mermaid* doll at the 70% level. Less improvement was obtained with the third (cup) symbol. Beth's highest level of performance in this third leg of the intervention was only 40%.

Overall, the results reported by Sutter and Demchak (2023) suggest that the intervention procedures were effective in increasing Beth's independent use of three tangible symbols. However, the relatively lower level of performance reached with the second and third trained symbols suggests lingering difficulties for her with respect to discriminating between the three symbols in the array. This may reflect the fact that the total amount of training provided to Beth was not extensive and decreased with each successive symbol. That is, Beth had 25 intervention sessions with the ball, 21 with the *Little Mermaid*, but only 11 with the cup symbol. It is also the case that modified intervention procedures were introduced at different points during intervention. For example, changes to the quality of social reinforcement started with the fifth intervention session on the ball, and the positioning prompt (i.e., moving the *Little Mermaid* symbol closer) started more than halfway through the intervention process on that second symbol (i.e., on the 13th session out of a total of 21 sessions). It is possible that continuing sessions using the final iteration of the intervention procedures would have enabled Beth to reach higher levels of proficiency. Alternatively, the relatively lower levels of performance with the second (*Little Mermaid*) and third (cup) symbols could suggest a reinforcement problem. Music, foods, and beverages might simply have been less powerful reinforcers for Beth than access to the ball. Perhaps incorporating preference assessments intermittently may have shed light on performance during training and possibly provided alternative items to be included in the instruction.

Indications for the Use of Tangible Symbols

Results of the intervention studies reviewed in this chapter suggest that tangible symbols can represent a viable communication strategy for nonverbal and minimally verbal people with severe disabilities. Rowland and Schweigert (2009) noted that tangible symbols may be indicated for "individuals who lack the communication skills to communicate clearly using speech or other abstract symbols systems, such as sign language" (p. 2). To these authors, the option of using tangible symbols may be indicated for a fairly wide range of nonverbal/minimally verbal people with intellectual, physical, and/or sensory impairments. Tangible symbols appear particularly well suited to individuals with significant vision impairment provided that the tangible symbols within a set can be distinguished from one another by touch and feel rather than visually. Such circumstances would tend to rule out communication systems using picture cards, photographs, or line drawings (see Chaps. 7 and 8). Tangible symbols may also be indicated for use by deafblind individuals (Sigafoos et al., 2008).

The research reviewed in this chapter provides a fair amount of experimental evidence to tentatively support the use of systematic instructional strategies for teaching nonverbal, visually impaired, and multiply handicapped individuals to use tangible symbols. However, Rowland and Schweigert (2009) noted the importance of considering existing communication abilities when assessing a person's candidacy for use of a tangible symbol system. Specifically, Rowland and Schweigert indicated that individuals who enter intervention with some existing level of prelinguistic or pre-symbolic communication ability (e.g., use of gestures and vocalizations) are likely to respond more quickly to intervention efforts aimed at teaching tangible symbols. On the other hand, Rowland and Schweigert (2000) reported success in teaching tangible symbol use to a relatively large and heterogeneous sample of children and adolescents who presented with "a wide range of abilities" (p. 72). In fact, 35 of the 41 participants in their study learned to request using tangible symbols. These positive findings from a relatively large sample suggest that tangible symbols may be indicated for use with people having widely differing types and levels of disability conditions, as well as differing communication abilities.

In most of the intervention studies reviewed in this chapter, participants were successfully taught to reach out, touch, pick up, and/or hand over tangible symbols as a means of making choices and/or requesting preferred objects and activities. As noted in Chap. 4, requesting is a priority intervention target in part because such skills enable the person to express wants and needs and exert some degree of control or self-determination over the environment (Johnston et al., 2012; Reichle et al., 1991). Similar rationale for teaching choice making have been offered (Shevin & Klein, 2004). Thus, teaching the functional use of tangible symbols for requesting and choice making might therefore be indicated as the initial communication objective for nonverbal/minimally verbal individuals with severe/multiple disabilities and significant vision impairment. The studies reviewed in this chapter also support the use of the Picture Exchange Communication System (Frost & Bondy, 2002) as a starting point for teaching the functional use of tangible symbols, specifically the teaching protocols associated with Phases 1 (i.e., initial exchange with an attending communication partner) and 2 (approaching/recruiting the attention of distant partners).

Rowland and Schweigert (2000, 2009) suggested that tangible symbol systems may provide a bridge toward the use of more abstract and formal communication strategies, such as speech, picture symbols, printed words, or the use of Braille for blind people. This suggestion is consistent with the more general observation that the direct manipulation of objects for communication purposes typically gives way as more complex language develops (Guevara & Rodŕiguez, 2023). Indeed, Rowland and Schweigert (2000) found that some students who learned to use tangible symbols through their intervention efforts were later "able to use abstract symbol systems" (p. 72).

Contraindications to the Use of Tangible Symbols

Tangible symbols are contraindicated for individuals who lack sufficient motors skills to select tangible symbols in some reliable and consistent manner. An effective selection response could thus be seen as a necessary prerequisite skill. An effective selection response is also generally seen as a necessary prerequisite to the use of other aided communication strategies (Reichle et al., 1991), such as the use of a picture-exchange communication strategy (Chap. 7) or a speech-generating device (Chap. 8). In the studies reviewed in this chapter, the selection responses being taught mainly consisted of reaching out and touching (or picking up) three-dimensional objects. In addition to reaching for, touching, and/or picking up a symbol, Rowland (1990) suggested that some individuals could learn to select tangible symbols by pointing to or looking at the symbol. Teaching tangible symbol use may be challenging if the person is unable to execute one or more such actions. Various assistive technology configurations may provide a means for individuals with limited motor skills to reliably select tangible or other types of aided communication symbols (see Chap. 9).

Lack of portability could become a potential disadvantage for users of tangible symbols. A set of three-dimensional tangible symbols, such as those illustrated in Figs. 6.1 and 6.2 for example, could quickly become cumbersome as the number of symbols in the set increases. Another potential disadvantage for users of tangible symbol systems stems from the fact that this method of communication is rather unique and thus may be less readily understood by unfamiliar listeners. This potential disadvantage might be overcome by training communication partners on how to interact with and respond to tangible symbol users. This type of partner training could be modeled on approaches that have been successfully applied to support the communicative partners of manual signers, for example, as discussed in Chap. 5.

Implementation Considerations

A factor that needs to be considered when designing a tangible symbol system is the type(s) of tangible symbols to teach. Most of the intervention studies reviewed in this chapter used three-dimensional real objects, miniature objects, or parts of real objects. And in most of these studies, the participants acquired functional use of the targeted symbols relatively quickly. However, rapid acquisition of tangible symbols may have more to do with the functional value of those symbols, rather than any inherent properties of the symbols themselves. That is, in most cases the tangible symbols were probably meaningful to the person because their use resulted in gaining access to highly preferred objects and activities. Acquisition of a tangible system might therefore be facilitated with symbols that closely resemble the person's preferences. While consideration of symbol transparency is important, the visible appearance of a symbol will be irrelevant to blind people. For these individuals, the more important feature is the extent to which symbols can be identified and discriminated on the basis of tactile cues (e.g., shape, size, and texture).

While it makes sense to consider symbols that are personally meaningful, some symbols may only become meaningful through intervention. That is, the communicative meaning or purpose of touching a miniature cup might emerge only after the child has been repeatedly prompted and reinforced for this response. Thus, meaningfulness could be seen as partly a function of how tangible symbols are taught. The most meaningful symbols may be those that, when used, are most likely to consistently result in a reinforcing consequence for the user.

The intervention studies reviewed in this chapter point to the value of structured intervention sessions with multiple learning opportunities. Given that requesting and choice making are often targeted for intervention, it would seem important to ensure opportunities occur when there is a need or motivation to communicate a request (Drasgow et al., 1999). Strategies for ensuring motivation and creating the need for requesting include (a) offering preferred items, (b) momentarily interrupting a preferred stimulus, (c) temporarily blocking access to a preferred object or activity, and (d) providing incomplete or small portions of a requested item (Sigafoos, 1999). In the intervention studies reviewed in this chapter, requesting opportunities were often created by presenting/offering preferred items. Nonvisual/nonverbal methods of signaling such offers may need to be devised for visually impaired and deafblind participants. A critical component of any teaching opportunity is ensuring that the correct communication response occurs so that it can then be reinforced. Initially, correct responding may have to be prompted, but ultimately prompts will need to be faded to promote spontaneity.

Summary and Conclusion

Tangible symbols typically consist of three-dimensional miniature objects or parts of objects that relate in some way to corresponding real-world referents. These types of tangible symbols may represent an effective communication strategy for some people with severe disabilities. The results of the studies reviewed in this chapter suggest that functional use of tangible symbols can be successfully taught using well-established systematic instructional procedures, including protocols associated with the Picture Exchange Communication System (Bondy & Frost, 1994, 1998; Frost & Bondy, 2002; Chap. 7). Most studies in this area have focused on teaching individuals to use tangible symbols to make choices and request preferred objects and activities. There has also been success in teaching individuals to use tangible symbols as tacts (e.g., naming responses) and to facilitate transitions.

Intervention to teach functional use of tangible symbols may be especially relevant to people with severe disabilities who are nonverbal and visually impaired because tangible symbols are permanent and concrete and can be discriminated via touch and feel. Contraindications include use with individuals who lack sufficient motor skills to physically manipulate or otherwise select (e.g., point, reach for, touch, and/or pick up) symbols. A potential disadvantage is that a tangible symbol system may become cumbersome as the number of symbols increases. Factors to consider when designing and implementing a tangible symbol system include the selection of tangible symbols and approaches for creating effective teaching opportunities.

References

Ali, E., MacFarland, S. Z., & Umbreit, J. (2011). Effectiveness of combining tangible symbols with the picture exchange communication system to teach requesting skills to children with multiple disabilities including visual impairment. *Education and Training in Autism and Developmental Disabilities, 46*(3), 425–435. https://doi.org/jstor.org/stable/23880596

Bondy, A. S., & Frost, L. A. (1994). The picture exchange communication system. *Focus on Autistic Behavior, 9*(3), 1–19.

Bondy, A. S., & Frost, L. A. (1998). The picture exchange communication system. *Seminars in Speech and Language, 19*(4), 373–388. https://doi.org/10.1055/s-2008-1064055

Cascella, P. W. (2014). Tangible object symbols: A case study with an adult with multiple disabilities. *Journal of Visual Impairment and Blindness, 108*(3), 249–253.

Drasgow, E., Halle, J. W., & Sigafoos, J. (1999). Teaching communication to learners with severe disabilities: Motivation, response competition, and generalisation. *Australasian Journal of Special Education, 23*(1), 47–63. https://doi.org/10.1017/S1030011200024507

Fried-Oken, M., Mooney, A., & Kinsella, M. (2019, February). Cognitive demands checklist for augmentative and alternative communication (CDC4AAC). Presentation at the Assistive Technology Industry Association (ATIA) Annual Conference, Orlando, FL. Retrieved September 25, 2024, from https://rerc-aac.psu.edu/2019/04/28/cognitive-demands-checklist-for-aac-fried-oken-et-al-2019/

Frost, L., & Bondy, A. S. (2002). *The picture exchange communication system training manual* (2nd ed.). Pyramid Educational Products.

Guevara, I., & Rodŕiguez, C. (2023). Developing communication through objects: Ostensive gestures as the first gestures in children's development. *Developmental Review, 68*, 1–26. https://doi.org/10.1016/j.dr.2023.101076

Ivy, S. E., Hatton, D. D., & Hooper, J. D. (2014). Using the picture exchange communication system with students with visual impairment. *Exceptional Children, 80*(4), 474–488. https://doi.org/10.1177/0014402914527239

Ivy, S. E., Robbins, A., & Kerr, M. G. (2020). Adapting the picture exchange communication system using tangible symbols for young learners with significant multiple disabilities. *Augmentative and Alternative Communication, 36*(3), 166–178. https://doi.org/10.1080/07434618.2020.1826051

Johnston, S. S., Reichle, J., Feeley, K. M., & Jones, E. A. (2012). *AAC strategies for individuals with moderate to severe disabilities*. Brookes Publishing Co.

Lund, S. K., & Troha, J. M. (2008). Teaching young people who are blind and have autism to make requests using a variation on the picture exchange communication system with tactile symbols: A preliminary investigation. *Journal of Autism and Developmental Disorders, 38*(4), 719–730. https://doi.org/10.1007/s10803-007-0439-4

Parker, A. T., Banda, D. R., Davidson, R. C., & Liu-Gitz, L. (2010). Adapting the picture exchange communication system for a student with visual impairment and autism: A case study. *AER Journal: Research and Practice in Visual Impairment and Blindness, 3*(1), 2–11.

Reichle, J., Beukelman, D. R., & Light, J. C. (2002). *Exemplary practices for beginning communicators*. Brookes Publishing Co.

Reichle, J., York, J., & Sigafoos, J. (1991). *Implementing augmentative and alternative communication: Strategies for learners with severe disabilities*. Brookes Publishing Co.

Roche, L., Sigafoos, J., Lancioni, G. L., O'Reilly, M. F., Green, V. A., Sutherland, D., van der Meer, L., Schlosser, R. W., Marschik, P. B., & Edrisinha, C. (2014a). Tangible symbols as an AAC option for individuals with developmental disabilities: A systematic review of intervention studies. *Augmentative and Alternative Communication, 30*(1), 28–39. https://doi.org/10.3109/07434618.2013.878958

Roche, L., Sigafoos, J., Lancioni, G. L., O'Reilly, M. F., van der Meer, L., Achmadi, D., Green, V. A., Kagohara, D., Sutherland, D., Rayner, C., & Marschik, P. B. (2014b). Comparing tangible symbols, picture exchange, and a direct selection response for enabling two boys with developmental disabilities to access preferred stimuli. *Journal of Developmental and Physical Disabilities, 26*(3), 249–261. https://doi.org/10.1007/s10882-013-9361-1

Rowland, C. (1990). *Tangible symbol systems: Symbolic communication for individuals with multisensory impairments*. Communication Skill Builders.

Rowland, C., & Schweigert, P. (1989). Tangible symbols: Symbolic communication for individuals with multisensory impairments. *Augmentative and Alternative Communication, 5*(4), 226–234. https://doi.org/10.1080/07434618912331275276

Rowland, C., & Schweigert, P. (2000). Tangible symbols, tangible outcomes. *Augmentative and Alternative Communication, 16*(2), 61–78. https://doi.org/10.1080/07434610012331278914

Rowland, C., & Schweigert, P. (2009). *Tangible symbol systems primer*. Retrieved September 24, 2024, from https://communicationmatrix.org/Community/Posts/Content/6624

Schlosser, R. W., Shane, H., Sorce, J., Loul, R., Bloomfield, E., Debrowski, L., DeLuca, T., Miller, S., Schneider, D., & Neff, A. (2012). Animation of graphic symbols representing verbs and prepositions: Effects on transparency, name agreement, and identification. *Journal of Speech, Language, and Hearing Research, 55*(2), 342–358. https://doi.org/10.1044/1092-4388(2011/10-0164)

Sevcik, R. A., Barton-Hulsey, A., Romski, M., & Hyatt Fonseca, A. (2018). Visual-graphic symbol acquisition in school age children with developmental and language delays. *Augmentative and Alternative Communication, 34*(4), 265–275. https://doi.org/10.1080/07434618.2018.1522547

Shevin, M., & Klein, N. K. (2004). The importance of choice-making skills for students with severe disabilities. *Research and Practice for Persons with Severe Disabilities, 29*(3), 161–168. https://doi.org/10.2511/rpsd.29.3.161

Sigafoos, J. (1999). Creating opportunities for augmentative and alternative communication: Strategies for involving people with developmental disabilities. *Augmentative and Alternative Communication, 15*(3), 183–190. https://doi.org/10.1080/07434619912331278715

Sigafoos, J., Didden, R., Schlosser, R., Green, V. A., O'Reilly, M. F., & Lancioni, G. E. (2008). A review of intervention studies on teaching AAC to individuals who are deaf and blind. *Journal of Developmental and Physical Disabilities, 20*(1), 71–99. https://doi.org/10.1007/s10882-007-9081-5

Sutter, C., & Demchak, M. (2023). Evaluation of the system of least prompts to teach symbol use to children who are deafblind. *Education and Training in Autism and Developmental Disabilities, 58*(3), 354–371.

Thistle, J. J., & Wilkinson, K. M. (2013). Working memory demands of aided augmentative and alternative communication for individuals with developmental disabilities. *Augmentative and Alternative Communication, 29*(3), 235–245. https://doi.org/10.3109/07434618.2013.815800

Trief, E. (2007). The use of tangible cues for children with multiple disabilities and visual impairment. *Journal of Visual Impairment and Blindness, 101*(10), 613–619. https://doi.org/10.1177/0145482X0710101006

Trief, E., Bruce, S. M., Cascella, P. W., & Ivy, S. (2009). The development of a universal tangible symbol system. *Journal of Visual Impairment and Blindness, 103*(7), 425–430. https://doi.org/10.1177/0145482X0910300706

Trief, E., Cascella, P. W., & Bruce, S. M. (2013). A field study of a standardized tangible symbol system for learners who are visually impaired and have multiple disabilities. *Journal of Visual Impairment & Blindness, 107*(3), 180–191. https://doi.org/10.1177/0145482X1310700303

Turnell, R., & Carter, M. (1994). Establishing a repertoire of requesting for a student with severe and multiple disabilities using tangible symbols and naturalistic time delay. *Australia and New Zealand Journal of Developmental Disabilities, 19*(3), 193–207.

Chapter 7
Effective Communication Using Picture Exchange

Introduction

Pictures and related types of communication symbols (e.g., line drawings, photographs) represent forms of aided augmentative and alternative communication (AAC) that have been widely used to support communication in nonverbal and minimally verbal individuals with severe disabilities. For example, pictures can be introduced to augment specific prelinguistic behaviors where a person is taught to point to a picture of an item (such as a favorite toy) rather than reach for the desired item, which is a type of prelinguistic communication response as described in Chap. 3. Pictures are also used to guide performance in relation to following daily schedules or activities (see Chap. 10). For example, at the beginning of a school day, a student is introduced to the upcoming classroom activities (e.g., circle time, followed by play, followed by reading, followed by nap time) with pictures of each activity presented in sequence on a laminated card. As each activity is completed the student removes the picture of that activity and is reminded of the next classroom activity. Such picture schedules can make the daily classroom structure more predictable, which can reduce challenging behaviors for students with severe disabilities (van Dijk & Gage, 2018). Possibly the most comprehensive picture-based system to support persons with severe disabilities is the Picture Exchange Communication System (PECS) developed by Bondy and Frost (2011).

PECS is a low-tech aided AAC system that was designed for persons who are nonverbal or experience speech and language delays. PECS is extensively used in clinical/educational settings with young autistic children (Alsayedhassan et al., 2016). The effectiveness of PECS has also received extensive attention in the research literature (Paris et al., 2024). PECS incorporates both developmental and behavioral perspectives in terms of how communication is conceptualized and how instructions with pictures are used to support communication (Bondy & Frost, 2011). To clarify, targeted communication goals follow a normative developmental

J. Sigafoos et al., *Communication Strategies for People with Severe Disabilities*, Autism and Child Psychopathology Series,
https://doi.org/10.1007/978-3-031-83807-1_7

sequence whereby the child is initially taught to request concrete items and gradually proceeds to more complicated communication goals, such as commenting on items/activities, and eventually communicating in sentences. However, instructional strategies (methods to teach targeted communication skills) and the specific communication skills themselves are couched in behavior-analytic terms. For example, mands and tacts (see Table 5.2) are used to describe requests and comments, respectively. In addition, the instructional technology used to teach PECS consists of evidence-based practices rooted in behavioral analysis (i.e., systematic instruction). This symbiosis of developmental and behavioral approaches is not unusual in comprehensive interventions for autistic children (see Lovaas, 1987, for an early example).

There are several facets of PECS that make it a popular AAC approach for autistic children and others with severe communication impairment. First, PECS is a manualized approach and the manual provides a detailed guide on how to implement the protocols. Also, the materials are commercially available (e.g., pictures and booklets) and are relatively inexpensive. Relatedly, pictures are relatively easy and inexpensive to create, adapt, and reproduce. For example, to enhance the iconicity of a picture, a photograph of the item may be taken (e.g., a favorite toy) and incorporated as a picture symbol to be used as part of the communication teaching program. This may be an advantage over other aided [high-tech] devices, which may be expensive and difficult for frontline staff to adapt, maintain, update, and program (see Chap. 8). Second, PECS is comprehensive in its approach to teaching communication—beginning with simple requests for preferred items and proceeding to more complicated social communication interchanges, such as commenting and expanding communication exchanges to complete sentences. Third, the instructional strategies used to teach PECS—such as preference assessment, programming generalization, systems of prompts, chaining, fading—are all evidence-based practices derived from decades of research in the field of applied behavior analysis (Brown et al., 2020). Many special education teachers, for example, would likely be familiar with these instructional strategies as they are the gold standard for teaching students with severe disabilities. Fourth, PECS does not require many precursor skills on the part of the communicator, such as making eye contact or joint attention skills. The communicator needs only to be able to retrieve and place a picture card in the hand of the listener for instruction to proceed. This starting point bodes well for early success when teaching communication skills.

PECS consists of six teaching phases that are designed to teach a functional communication repertoire to the student. In Phase 1, the student is taught to exchange a picture for a desired item. Prior to training trials, a preference assessment is conducted to identify a hierarchy of preferred items for the child. Next, the child is taught to engage in a communicative exchange with a listener to achieve access to the desired item. This is accomplished by placing the desired item close to, but not within reach of, the student. The student may then engage in reaching or some other behavior to access the preferred item. At this point, a trainer physically guides the student to pick up a picture or photograph of the item and place it in the hand of a second person (the listener). The listener then gives the student immediate access to the requested item while also verbally naming the item that the student has just requested. The communicative act involves the selection of the picture and the exchange of the picture for the preferred item. It is important to note that training trials initially involve two individuals (i.e., a trainer and a listener) in addition to the student. The trainer physically prompts the communication of the student (i.e., prompts the student to pick up and place the picture in the listener's hand). The listener is the person who acknowledges and responds to the communication of the student. During training trials in Phase 1, the trainer gradually fades physical prompts until the student independently (without prompts) picks up the picture and places it in the hand of the listener when the desired item is physically available. It is recommended that generalization of this new requesting response be actively programmed for from the beginning of training. This can be accomplished by using different trainers, listeners, preferred items, and contexts (see Stokes & Baer, 1977, for an overview of the strategies to facilitate generalization).

Phase 2 builds upon the manding (requesting) skills learned in Phase 1. In a sense, Phase 2 is designed to make the new requesting repertoire established in Phase 1 more resilient and persistent when faced with everyday obstacles. For example, the student may have to travel across a room or even to another location to find the listener and deliver the picture card. The listener may also appear distracted (with their back to the student) when the student attempts to communicate, thus necessitating the need for the student to first gain the listener's attention. Additionally, during Phase 2, the student is taught to locate the picture card when the desired item is presented. For example, during some trials the student is taught to go to a location (e.g., a specific drawer, or a cabinet) to access the picture card and then present the card to the listener prior to receiving access to the requested item. The picture card is also presented on the front page of a binder in the latter part of Phase 2 training. This is to introduce the student to a binder that will be useful as the student's set of picture vocabulary increases. Again, in Phase 2 the trainer is present and uses physical prompts to facilitate successful performance of the targeted skills. Prompting is again gradually faded until the student masters the skills independently. Generalization is also actively programmed across trainers, listeners, preferred items, and contexts.

During Phase 3, students are now taught to discriminate between pictures of items. At the beginning of Phase 3, the student is presented with a nondesired and a highly desired item simultaneously while corresponding picture cards of these items are in front of the student. As in previous phases, it is critical to clearly determine the preferred and nonpreferred (or neutral) status of items via a systematic preference assessment prior to implementing instruction aimed at teaching requesting. If the student chooses the preferred item (by selecting the picture card of the preferred item from the front of the manual and placing it in the hand of the listener), then the listener immediately gives the preferred item coupled with verbal praise. Positive acknowledgment for choosing the correct picture (e.g., verbal praise) is given prior to the student exchanging the card with the listener. If the student exchanges the card depicting the neutral item, then they are given the neutral item. Error correction procedures are then initiated and include returning items to their original location as at the beginning of the trial, the trainer pointing to the picture card of the preferred item and physically prompting the student to select the picture of the preferred item, and verbal praise for selecting the correct picture. During error correction procedures, the student does not get access to the preferred item. Following error correction, a discrimination trial is then repeated.

Once discrimination between pictures representing preferred versus neutral items is achieved, then the student is taught to discriminate between two preferred items. During these training trials, when the student exchanges a card, the student is presented with both items and instructed to *Take it*. If the student takes the item corresponding to the card presented to the listener, then they can engage with the item. However, if they choose the other item (the noncorresponding item), then error correction procedures, as described above, are implemented. The number of picture cards and items is increased gradually during Phase 3 until there are approximately six picture cards and corresponding items simultaneously available during each training trial. Mastered skills from Phases 1 and 2 are interspersed during Phase 3 to solidify performance and provide opportunities for successful performance and positive consequences.

Phase 4 is implemented once the student is successfully discriminating between groups of pictures to request items and when these requesting skills are occurring across multiple contexts and persons (i.e., when the skills have generalized). Phase 4 consists of expanding to multisymbol requests. For example, the student is taught (via the same systematic instruction procedures described in the earlier phases of PECS) to construct a two-picture sentence with the phrase *"I want"* placed before the picture of the desired item. The student places both pictures on a sentence strip (e.g., *"I want"* and *"firetruck"*) and then hands the strip to the listener. The listener reads the strip aloud in an animated approving tone and delivers the requested item to the student. Again, Phase 4 builds upon earlier phases with discrimination opportunities and instruction occurring across a variety of persons and contexts. Trials incorporating the goals of earlier phases are interspersed periodically to provide practice using earlier learned skills, which should facilitate maintenance.

In Phase 5, the student is taught to answer a direct question from the listener, such as *What do you want?* The student is prompted to answer the question using a sentence frame and then receives the desired item. A progressive time delay instructional protocol is used whereby the listener asks, *What do you want?* and then immediately gestures to the "*I want*" card. The child then completes the two-picture phrase ("*I want*" and "*apple*") and hands the phrase to the listener. Finally, the listener gives the desired item to the student. The gestural prompt to respond to the listener's question is gradually delayed until the student spontaneously produces the two-picture phrase when asked, *What do you want?* Programming for maintenance and generalization is also incorporated in the phase.

In the final phase (Phase 6), the student is taught to comment. Commenting on items and activities can be difficult to teach to some nonverbal individuals with severe disabilities. For example, prelinguistic forms of requesting (Chap. 3) are evident in young autistic children, hence the focus in Phases 1–5 on teaching requesting and responding to questions regarding desired items/activities. Commenting, in contrast to requesting, serves a different more social communicative function and that is sharing a perspective with the listener. The skills taught in Phases 1–5, such as constructing phrases and spontaneously responding to questions, are considered foundational to teaching the commenting skills targeted in Phase 6. In Phase 6, phrases such as "*I see*" or "*What is it?*" are gradually introduced to the student's communication board. For example, an item is made visible and the student is prompted to select the "*I see*" card. A progressive time delay procedure is used to teach the student to spontaneously select the "*I see*" and picture of the item presented and give to the listener. The listener responds with an animated acknowledgment that they also see the item. In commenting trials, the student does not receive the item as a consequence to distinguish this skill from a mand or request. However, requesting (Phase 5) and commenting trials are interspersed during Phase 6 to develop the student ability to discriminate between commenting and requesting. Maintenance and generalization are actively programmed throughout the day.

PECS is an ongoing communication process where additional requesting and commenting phrases are added over the course of intervention to expand the student's repertoire. Additional target concepts include responses to further specify communication responses, such as by color ("*I see*" "*green dinosaur*") or shape ("*I want*" "*round cookie*").

Review of PECS Intervention Studies

An extensive amount of research has been conducted over the past few decades to evaluate the effectiveness of teaching PECS to nonverbal and minimally verbal individuals with severe disabilities. Most of this research has focused on teaching PECS to young autistic children. For example, in a recent literature review, Paris et al. (2024) summarized the effectiveness of 49 intervention studies published in peer-reviewed journals. Overall, Paris et al. concluded that PECS is an effective approach for teaching students to exchange pictures to communicate requests. However, there are limitations to this research. For example, very little research has taught all PECS phases. Also, the experimental rigor of many of these published studies has been critiqued (Preston & Carter, 2009). To illustrate this research literature, a selective review of six studies is presented below. Three of the studies described below were conducted in home settings and three in school settings. The six studies described in this section are summarized in Table 7.1 according to settings, participants, intervention, and outcomes.

Table 7.1 Summary of six PECS intervention studies with learners with severe communication needs

Study	Setting	Participants	Intervention	Outcome
Adkins and Axelrod (2001)	Special education classroom	1 student (aged 7 years) with pervasive developmental disorder	Adapted PECS training with generalization probes	Rapid acquisition, generalization, and spontaneous use of PECS (Phases 1–3)
Ganz et al. (2005)	Home setting	1 child (aged 5 years) with severe autism	Adapted PECS protocol using tangible symbols	Child acquired PECS Phases 1 and 3
Gordon et al. (2011)	School settings	84 autistic school children	Teachers taught to implement all PECS phases	Increased spontaneous communication with higher functioning students making most progress
Hill and Flores (2014)	Extended school year program	5 students. 3 preschool (3–4 years old). 2 elementary (both 9 years old)	Comparison of PECS delivered via iPad versus physical pictures during snack time	3 students achieved Phase 5 of PECS
Park et al. (2011)	Home settings	3 mother–child dyads. Children were 2–3 years old and had autism	Modeling, roleplay, feedback, and video vignettes to teach mothers to train PECS Phases 1–3	Mothers successfully implemented Phases 1–3 with corresponding increases in child communication
Schreibman and Stahmer (2014)	In home and clinical setting	19 parent–child dyads. All children were diagnosed with autism (aged 20–45 months)	Parent–child dyads trained in PECS in clinic with in-home follow-up	12 of the 19 children completed all PECS phases and parents were satisfied with the program

Examples of PECS Research Conducted in the Home

An interesting study by Ganz et al. (2005) sought to teach PECS to an autistic child in the home setting. The child (pseudo name Elsie) was 5 years old at the time of the study. A battery of assessments revealed that Elsie functioned in the severe autism range per the *Childhood Autism Rating Scale* (Schopler et al., 1988) and exhibited severe developmental delay with a developmental score of 9 months per the *Psychoeducational Profile Revised* (Schopler et al., 1990). Elsie had not mastered any pre-academic tasks such as coloring, stacking, or sorting. She was observed to communicate predominantly through reaching and crying. She reportedly had no words and rarely made eye contact. The intervention was conducted by the experimenters in two areas of Elsie's home: a play area and the kitchen.

PECS training sessions lasted approximately 15 min, and there were 10 training trials per session. Training began with a preference assessment per the PECS training protocol. Elsie's mother and therapist were interviewed to determine a list of preferred stimuli (e.g., foods and toys). These items were then presented to Elsie using a multiple stimulus with replacement preference assessment protocol (Kang et al., 2013). Phase 1 of the PECS was then implemented; however, Elsie was unable to independently learn (without prompts) to exchange pictures for preferred items. Phase 1 was then adapted (Phase 1A) where Elsie was taught to touch a clear box containing a preferred item (which was placed in front of her). In other words, Elsie was taught to touch the box containing a preferred item and then received that item from the trainer. Once she reached criterion in Phase 1A, then a picture of the item was attached to the clear box containing the item and Elsie was successfully taught to exchange the box for the preferred item with the listener (Phase 1B). Training then progressed to Phase 3 where Elsie was taught to discriminate between the box with the picture attached and containing a preferred item versus a box containing a nonpreferred item. The Phase 3 protocol adhered to the procedures outlined by Bondy and Frost (2011). Finally, in Phase 3, the clear boxes were removed and Elsie successfully discriminated between picture cards to access preferred items from the listener.

Ganz et al. (2005) describe the procedure in this study as a modified version of the PECS protocol. The rationale for modification of the manualized procedures is compelling in this case. That is, because Elsie did not master the skills of PECS Phase 1, the authors aimed to enhance the iconicity of the stimuli by pairing the picture symbols with a clear box containing the item represented in the picture and by teaching Elsie to exchange the box plus picture for the preferred item. The authors did not include Phase 2 training as part of the intervention as it was estimated that generalizing and persisting with the requesting response would be too difficult for Elsie. The researchers note that the intervention goal was to equip Elsie and her parents with basic requesting and choice-making skills. It took almost 100 teaching sessions (with 10 trials per session) for Elsie to master PECS Phases 1 and 3. This important case study by Ganz et al. is a clear example that not all of the phases described in the PECS manual are likely to be relevant to all intervention candidates. However, with expert clinical guidance the PECS protocol may be successfully adapted (as in the case of Elsie) to promote acquisition of picture-based functional communication skills.

Park et al. (2011) conducted the first study that sought to teach mothers to implement PECS with their young autistic children in the home setting. Given that parents are usually the primary carers for these young children, it is critical that they are involved in teaching and supporting communication skills. Evaluating training protocol to effectively teach parents to use evidence-based communication strategies is therefore a priority. Three mothers were taught to use PECS with their children. Parent training and evaluation of PECS outcomes were implemented individually with each parent–child dyad in their respective homes. All children were between 2 and 3 years of age. None of the children or parents had prior experience using PECS. The children had limited or no language and their primary means of requesting involved prelinguistic acts, such as pointing or leading an adult to a preferred item. None of the children exhibited any serious challenging behavior. One child was diagnosed in the mild–moderate range, while the other two were scored as having severe autism per the *Childhood Autism Rating Scale* (Schopler et al., 1988).

Mothers were taught to implement Phases 1–3 of PECS with their children. Prior to each phase, the mothers were familiarized with materials (e.g., picture cards, booklets) and taught to implement the instructional procedures for that phase through written instructions, modeling, roleplay, and feedback from a trainer. Mothers also reviewed a video clip of models performing various types of responses during each phase. That is, each of these videos (one video per phase) showed a child engaged in the correct response, not responding, or responding incorrectly and the trainer responding appropriately as per the PECS training protocol. The PECS protocols for Phases 1–3 were implemented with very little modification from the manualized versions. The procedures included ongoing preference assessment during the training and tests for acquisition, generalization, and maintenance of the newly learned communication skills. One notable aspect of the training included a baseline condition that assessed the child's ability to communicate with the cards prior to any training. In the baseline condition, the mother sat across from the child at a table. Two pictures of preferred items were placed in front of the child and the mother presented the two preferred items. The child was given access to the preferred item if they selected and exchanged a picture card with the mother or if they used a prelinguistic communicative response, such as reaching. None of the children used the pictures to request preferred items during this baseline condition. Another notable aspect of this research is the use of a procedural integrity measure to assess whether the mother was implementing the PECS protocol with accuracy. The experimenters used a checklist (specific to each training phase) to assess whether the mother was implementing the protocol accurately. Procedural integrity was assessed for at least 61% of randomly selected sessions across all participants.

Overall, the results of this research by Park et al. (2011) provided a convincing demonstration of the effectiveness of training parents to implement the PECS with children in the home. All three children acquired the communication skills for each of the three PECS phases. They also showed generalization and maintenance of these skills. Skill acquisition was a little slower for the two children with more severe levels of autistic symptoms. Child word utterances (clearly saying the name of a requested item) and word approximations (a vocalization that included at least one consonant and one vowel) were also measured during training—with little discernable change during the study. This reflects similar findings from other studies that have shown limited increases in vocalizations during PECS intervention (e.g., Anderson et al., 2007). All three mothers learned to accurately implement the PECS teaching protocol and used these protocols with a high degree of fidelity during teaching sessions. The authors employed changing criterion designs for each parent–child dyad to demonstrate experimental control. The ultimate veracity of this design is somewhat challenged because the dependent measure across each criterion phase is different (reflecting the skills taught during each separate phase of PECS). Following the study, the mothers completed a social validity survey that consisted of a series of questions to determine whether they found the procedures, goals, and outcomes of the PECS intervention acceptable. All mothers were positive about the teaching procedures and communication outcomes obtained with their child. Such positive social validity findings would predict that parents would continue to use the PECS following the study.

Most PECS studies have utilized single-case research designs to evaluate the effects of intervention on individual or small groups of participants. While single-case designs are an appropriate method for demonstrating functional relations between treatment and outcome, they are limited in terms of determining generalized assumptions of treatment effects. Preston and Carter (2009) called for the increased use of randomized control trials (RTCs) to determine the external validity of PECS. Along these lines, Schreibman and Stahmer (2014) compared the effects of pivotal response training (PRT; see Table 3.2) versus PECS on the development of communication/language using an RCT design. In this study, a total of 39 families across two research sites were recruited and randomly assigned to either PECS or PRT treatment conditions. All children (5 females and 34 males) were diagnosed with autism and were aged between 20 and 45 months at the beginning of treatment. A total of 19 children (plus their primary caregiver) were assigned to the PECS treatment condition.

The PECS intervention was delivered in clinic and home settings. Overall, children received about 258 hours of treatment over a 6-month period. Specifically, during the first 15 weeks, parent–child dyads attended two, 2-hour sessions weekly at a clinic where they were taught to implement PECS procedures. During these sessions, parents were trained to implement the PECS protocols through modeling, roleplay, and feedback by doctoral-level therapists. Additionally, trained therapists (undergraduate students) delivered five, 2-hour PECS teaching sessions in the home. For the final 8 weeks of treatment, parent–child dyads attended one, 2-hour training session at the clinic while in-home therapists delivered two, 2-hour sessions per week.

A series of standardized measures of spoken language, spoken vocabulary, and adaptive communication were administered before intervention, upon intervention completion, and during a follow-up assessment. The extent to which participants successfully mastered the various PECS phases and the degree of parental satisfaction with the program were also obtained following the intervention. Also, 12 of the 19 children in the PECS condition successfully completed all six phases of the protocol. Additionally, children who reached Phase 4 or higher demonstrated increases in spoken language. And children who successfully completed Phase 6 showed the strongest increases in spoken language. Parents also expressed satisfaction with the PECS intervention protocols. While the positive results of this study are impressive, some cautions may be warranted. The intervention intensity (involving over 200 hours of therapy across 23 weeks) may be impractical (both financially and in terms of time commitment) for many families. The RCT design used in this study did not include a no-treatment control condition (i.e., a matched group of children not assigned to a treatment condition). In fact, children in the second intervention group (i.e., the PRT group) also showed spoken language gains and there were no statistically significant differences between the PECS and PRT conditions.

Finally, severity of disability for each of the children was not described. It seems plausible that severity of the disability may influence intervention outcomes.

Examples of PECS Research Conducted in Schools

In an early and classic example of PECS intervention research, Adkins and Axelrod (2001) compared the effects of American Sign Language (ASL) (see Chap. 5) with PECS for teaching a child to mand/request preferred items. This child was a 7-year-old boy diagnosed with pervasive developmental disorder and ADHD. The student did not have any spontaneous words, but could imitate a few words and phrases. He also engaged in a variety of problem behaviors, such as aggression and elopement. Prior to the study, he received communication training using PECS and was reported to have learned 10–15 symbols.

The PECS procedures were conducted in the child's classroom during regular school hours. Training was implemented by an experimenter and sessions were conducted at a classroom table with the student and experimenter sitting across from one another. The experimenter offered a preferred object, which was placed out of the child's reach. The experimenter then guided the child's hand to pick up the correct picture (from an array of about 3–5 pictures) and place it in the experimenter's outstretched hand. Physical guidance was faded following six trials and the session continued until the student independently selected and presented the correct picture five consecutive times. Each session could consist of up to 40 training trials or until the training criterion was met.

An alternating treatment design was used to compare the efficiency of PECS training versus ASL with this student. Results showed that PECS produced more rapid acquisition of requests than ASL with PECS requiring about half the number of training trials to learn new requests. Two forms of generalization test were also incorporated within the study to assess learning outside of the training situation. On the same day and following a training session, a generalization test condition was conducted. In this generalization test, the preferred objects trained earlier in the day were presented, but without prompts. A second generalization condition was also conducted, which involved presenting requesting opportunities throughout the day during regular classroom activities. Overall, the results show rapid acquisition of new requests using the PECS system, strong generalization of requests, and spontaneous emission of requests throughout the day. However, these results must be interpreted with caution for several reasons. The study was conducted with only a single individual and therefore broad interpretations of the findings are not possible. In addition, the PECS training protocol used in this study deviated somewhat from the training protocol described by Bondy and Frost (2011). Also, critical aspects of the intervention were not described in sufficient detail to enable replication, such as details regarding how and when the preference assessments were conducted. Additionally, the intervention in this study focused on Phase 3 (discrimination training) with no information on training procedures or data for Phases 1 and 2.

Hill and Flores (2014) compared the standard low-tech version of PECS to a higher-tech version in which the PECS approach was configured for use with an iPad® equipped with Proloquo2Go® software (see Chap. 8). Participants included five students. Three of the students were preschoolers (age range 3–4 years), whereas the other two were of elementary school age (both 9 years). All students exhibited significant communication delays and were candidates for an aided communication intervention. Three of the students were diagnosed as having autism and two with developmental delay. The students attended extended school year services at a university-based program where this research took place. Classrooms consisted of 4–8 students with similar disabilities.

PECS intervention occurred during snack times during which students were offered a selection of three snacks and a drink. During PECS Phases 1 and 2, a therapist sat behind the students and acted as prompter while the teacher (acting as the listener) sat in front of the student, presented the snack items, and responded to student initiations. No preference assessments were conducted during the intervention, but it was assumed that the snacks were highly preferred. Additionally, PECS training was limited to the context of sitting at a table during snack time, potentially limiting generalization of the communication responses across stimuli and time. The higher-tech, iPad® version of PECS was also shown to be an effective strategy. The authors suggested using PECS in the low-tech form prior to introducing the higher-tech iPad® version because this may represent a more effective progression for some students with autism and other developmental disabilities.

An alternating treatment design was used for each student to compare the efficacy of PECS training versus the iPad®-based intervention. Additionally, interobserver reliability was conducted for student responding while treatment integrity was assessed by the prompter and listener. Three of the students achieved the skills associated with Phase 5 of the PECS protocol. That is, in response to the question *What do you want?*, they could independently construct a multipicture communication response using sentence strip (e.g., "*I want*" "*animal crackers*"), and hand to the teacher. One student failed to acquire the targeted exchanges due to limited fine motor skills. Another student began to use words appropriately to make request early and therefore did not require an aided communication strategy.

Gordon et al. (2011) sought to examine the form and function of spontaneous communication among 84 students who received teacher-implemented PECS training. Specifically, Gordon et al. sought to determine whether the use of PECS generalized beyond the treatment conditions to regular school routines and whether there were increases in spoken language during these school routines. Additionally, the authors sought to explore the relation between the level of severity of autism and changes in spontaneous communication following PECS training.

The study involved an RCT with three groups: an immediate, a delayed, and a no-treatment group. The PECS intervention was staggered across the immediate and delayed intervention groups, thereby maximizing the number of students exposed to the intervention and allowing for the assessment of maintenance effects for the immediate treatment group. To assess spontaneous communication during regular school routines, each student was videotaped (for 15 min) during regular snack periods on three occasions (prior to intervention and then following intervention on two more occasions over a 20-month period). Snack time was selected as it was likely to provide opportunities for both requesting and socializing. Frequency of child communication was measured including modality (e.g., picture exchange or use of vocalization or words) and communicative function (e.g., requesting or commenting).

Results of this study indicated that children increased in their use of pictures, vocalizations, and combinations of pictures and vocalizations to communicate following PECS training. Most communication initiations were related to requesting items, which may relate to the fact that observations were conducted at snack times when opportunities for requesting would likely have been frequent and the fact that social communication may be more difficult and/or less motivating for children with autism. Finally, less severe autistic symptomology at intervention onset tended to predict better communication outcomes for children.

In summary, a substantial amount of research has been published over the past 30 years that has demonstrated that picture-based systems, and in particular PECS, are viable communication strategies for nonverbal and minimally verbal people with severe disabilities. However, most of this communication intervention research has focused on teaching PECS to young autistic children. This is not surprising as PECS was designed to facilitate communication skills for this population. The studies summarized in Table 7.1 and described in this section suggest that children with autism can be taught to exchange pictures to request items and in some cases to engage in social commentary. Indeed, all of the children in the studies described in this section showed some increases in the targeted picture-based communication skills. Research has demonstrated that such interventions can be implemented in natural community settings and successfully delivered by parents and teachers.

Indications for Teaching PECS

There are several potential advantages and indications for use of picture exchange (particularly PECS) as an aided communication strategy for nonverbal and minimally verbal people with severe disabilities. Clinically, the use of pictures to support activity schedules, prompt skill development, and enable communication in nonverbal and minimally verbal people with severe disabilities is widespread in schools, daily activity centers, and community living arrangements. PECS has been extensively researched and widely recommended as a communication strategy for autistic children with minimal or no speech. Despite limitations in this research (e.g., few RCTs, limited assessment of maintenance and/or generalization, and limited treatment fidelity reported), most participants included in this research have, at a minimum, been successfully taught to spontaneously request preferred items via the exchange of pictures.

Several advantages of using PECS can be identified. PECS is a manualized procedure designed to teach an array of communication skills beginning with simple requesting of preferred items to engaging in social commentary. Bondy and Frost (2011) have clearly delineated instructional strategies for each of their six intervention phases, and these procedures have been successfully applied by therapists, parents, and teachers. This manualized approach might facilitate more consistent implementation. Relatedly, the instructional strategies used to teach communication exchange (e.g., preference assessments, time delay, physical guidance, prompt fading) have been extensively researched and can be considered evidence-based instructional practices. The materials used to teach communication (picture cards, manuals) are inexpensive to produce and easy to duplicate or develop to enable individualization.

The communication format used in PECS focuses on teaching the student to exchange pictures with a listener, which therefore could be seen as perhaps encouraging some more active engagement in communication exchange between student and listener. Such interactive responding may help ameliorate some of the key difficulties of autism, such as limited social interaction and joint attention. There do not appear to be any major cognitive precursor skills, such as the ability to match items, which means there is no need to delay beginning a PECS intervention. Relatedly, as students are initially taught to make requests for highly preferred items, successful learning of the initial exchange tends to occur quickly. There is some evidence to suggest that teaching PECS may facilitate spoken language contrary to some suggestions that an aided communication strategy may inhibit language development in people who are nonverbal or minimally verbal. PECS instruction seems to have a more facilitative effect on the emergence of natural speech production as students master the later phases (Phases 4–6) of PECS.

Contraindications for Teaching PECS

Some students may have such severe learning difficulties that they require an adapted training protocol. For example, in the study by Ganz et al. (2005), the student was unable to perform Phase 1 of training. In such situations, training protocols may need to be modified, as in the case of Ganz et al., where the picture plus the preferred item (visible in a transparent and sealed container) were paired to facilitate learning. Gradually, this student made progress through several phases of PECS. Many students with severe disabilities and limited communication ability may engage in problem behaviors, such as self-injury, property destruction, and aggression. These behaviors may be difficult to manage during PECS instruction and may need supplementary support plans, such as functional communication training (where the student is taught to use appropriate communication to replace problem behavior) as part of overall instructional programming. There is some research to indicate that PECS may mitigate some problem behavior (Charlop-Christy et al., 2002).

Another potential contraindication relates to students with physical impairments, which may make it difficult for them to perform the motor skills required for functional use of a picture-exchange communication strategy (e.g., pick up and deliver a picture card to the listener). For these individuals, some type of assistive access technology (e.g., a microswitch or sensor technology) might be indicated (see Chap. 9).

Implementing PECS requires personnel and skill resources. Phases 1 and 2 of PECS require two persons to be simultaneously present with the student (i.e., one person to prompt the student and another person to act as the listener). In many situations, such as the home, it may be impractical to expect two people to be simultaneously involved in such training with a student. Instructional protocols used to teach PECS—such as preference assessments, prompting, and fading—can be complicated for some communicative partners and may require some direct training and practice to master. Introductory workshops, as recommended by Bondy and Frost (2011), may be indicated to enable parents, teachers, and therapists to successfully implement the PECS protocols. In addition, some therapists, teachers, and parents may require additional training and follow-up observations plus feedback from trained specialists as each PECS phase arises in order to be able to implement the teaching procedures properly. This type of training and follow-up support may be difficult to achieve in some settings. However, technology such as tele-diagnosis and tele-assessment may be helpful as a way of supplementing direct mentoring.

Implementation Considerations

Several factors should be considered when implementing PECS. PECS is designed as a strategy to enhance communication for people who are nonverbal and minimally, but most research has focused on students with autism. Many students involved in this research have successfully learned to exchange pictures with a listener to access preferred items. Several studies have also reported that students can progress to more advanced PECS phases after learning to make the initial requesting exchange. PECS may be implemented even with students who lack certain cognitive skills, such as the ability to match real objects to pictures and in fact it is possible that such skills may develop as a result of participation in PECS training. PECS does not appear to inhibit natural speech production and may even have some facilitate effects in relation to speech. PECS may also have a positive impact on problem behavior, particularly if the function of the person's picture exchanges matches the function of their problem behavior.

The characteristics of the individual student must be considered when implementing PECS. People with more severe disabilities may require more intensive instruction to acquire skills and may not progress through all the phases of PECS. Much of the research presented in this chapter demonstrated that many people progress successfully to Phase 3 of PECS. This may be the case because the first three phases focus on teaching requests for preferred items, whereas the later phases of PECS target more social communication skills, which may not be inherently reinforcing to some individuals, such as autistic students. However, accurately discriminating and requesting preferred items is a laudable communication goal for many nonverbal and minimally verbal people with severe disabilities. Some candidates for picture-exchange systems and PECS training may require program modifications, such as enhancing the iconicity of the pictures, to facilitate learning. People who exhibit problem behaviors may require supplemental supports (e.g., functional communication training) as such behaviors may interfere with learning. Also, students with limited motor skills may require supplemental assistive technology (e.g., microswitches, sensors to capture purposive movements) to support their learning (see Chap. 9).

The technology used with PECS (e.g., picture cards, photographs, booklets, and word strips) is relatively inexpensive and easy to produce or duplicate. However, the instructional strategies used to successfully teach PECS may require a fair degree of training and practice in order for teachers, therapists, and parents to implement the instructional procedures successfully. It is important that those who implement PECS, such as teachers and parents, are adequately trained to implement these procedures and receive expert follow-up and support in criterion settings such as the home and/or school. Phases 1 and 2 of PECS require two trainers (i.e., a prompter and a listener) to be simultaneously available, which may be beyond the resources of some schools and homes. Ultimately, for PECS to be successful it must be programmed throughout the day and across persons, settings, and activities. Preference assessments must be conducted frequently (many times per day) to avoid satiation and identify possible novel preferred items/activities to be incorporated into instruction. Successful PECS instruction may require intensive input from those who are directly supporting the student.

Summary and Conclusion

Pictures and related types of communication symbols (e.g., line drawings, photographs) represent a widely used form of aided and low-tech forms of AAC. PECS is a manualized and empirically supported approach to teaching picture exchange-based communication skills to nonverbal and minimally verbal people. Most of the supporting research has to date involved students with autism. In the PECS program, the person is first taught to exchange pictures with a listener as a means of requesting preferred objects. Training then proceeds to discriminate between preferred/nonpreferred items, engaging in social commentary, and constructing multi-picture sentences. PECS training protocols make use of evidence-based instructional tactics derived from behavior-analytic research and principles. While the technology of PECS (e.g., picture cards, folders, sentence strips) is readily accessible, teaching a child to use PECS often requires systematic/structured intervention and ongoing monitoring and support from trained therapists.

Research examining the use of PECS is extensive, particularly with young autistic children. Overall findings from the research indicate that most children can successfully learn to use PECS to request preferred items and discriminate between preferred and nonpreferred items. Much of the research has not examined teaching the later phases of PECS, which involve social commenting and communicating in full sentences. This may be because autistic students find social commentary less reinforcing than communicating for preferred tangible items. Students with less severe autistic symptomology tend to respond better, with many learning to comment and complete full and complex sentences using picture cues. While the findings are limited, there is some evidence to indicate that students who begin PECS with some spoken vocabulary will show an increase in the production of spoken words during the later phases of training. However, students with more severe disabilities may require more intensive instruction, and may benefit from adaptations to the instructional protocol, such as by initially learning to exchange or reach for tangible symbols and then shaping these into line drawings/picture symbols.

References

Adkins, T., & Axelrod, S. (2001). Topography-versus selection-based responding: Comparison of mand acquisitions in each modality. *The Behavior Analyst Today, 2*(3), 259–266.

Alsayedhassan, B., Banda, D. R., & Griffin-Shirley, N. (2016). A review of picture exchange communication interventions implemented by parents and practitioners. *Child & Family Behavior Therapy, 38*(3), 191–208. https://doi.org/10.1080/07317107.2016.1203135

Anderson, A., Moore, D. W., & Bourne, T. (2007). Functional communication and other concomitant behavior change following PECS training: A case study. *Behaviour Change, 24*(3), 173–181. https://doi.org/10.1375/bech.24.3.173

Bondy, A. S., & Frost, L. A. (2011). *A picture's worth: PECS and other visual communication strategies in autism* (2nd ed.). Woodbine House.

Brown, F. E., McDonnell, J., & Snell, M. (2020). *Instruction of students with severe disabilities* (9th ed.). Pearson.

Charlop-Christy, M. H., Carpenter, M., Le, L., LeBlanc, L. A., & Kellet, K. (2002). Using the picture exchange communication system (PECS) with children with autism: Assessment of PECS acquisition, speech, social-communicative behavior, and problem behavior. *Journal of Applied Behavior Analysis, 35*(3), 213–231. https://doi.org/10.1901/jaba.2002.35-213

Ganz, J. B., Cook, K. E., Corbin-Newsome, J., Bourgeois, B., & Flores, M. (2005). Variations on the use of a pictorial alternative communication system with a child with autism and developmental delays. *Teaching Exceptional Children Plus, 1*(6), 3. http://escholarship.bc.edu/education/tecplus/vol1/iss6/3

Gordon, K., Pasco, G., McElduff, F., Wade, A., Howlin, P., & Charman, T. (2011). A communication-based intervention for nonverbal children with autism: What changes? Who benefits? *Journal of Consulting and Clinical Psychology, 79*(4), 447–457. https://doi.org/10.1037/a0024379. PMID: 21787048.

Hill, D. A., & Flores, M. M. (2014). Comparing the picture exchange communication system and the iPad for communication of students with autism spectrum disorder and developmental delay. *TechTrends, 58*(3), 45–53. https://doi.org/10.1007/s11528-014-0751-8

Kang, S., O'Reilly, M. F., Lancioni, G. E., Falcomata, T., Sigafoos, J., & Xu, H. (2013). Comparison of the predicative validity and consistency among preference assessment procedures: A review of the literature. *Research in Developmental Disabilities, 34*(4), 1125–1133. https://doi.org/10.1016/j.ridd.2012.12.021

Lovaas, O. I. (1987). Behavioral treatment and normal educational and intellectual functioning in young autistic children. *Journal of Consulting and Clinical Psychology, 55*(1), 3–9. https://doi.org/10.1037/0022-006X.55.1.3

Paris, A., Denne, L. D., Grindle, C. F., May, R., Apanasionok, M. M., & Hastings, R. P. (2024). Facilitators and barriers to the implementation of the picture exchange communication system (PECS): A systematic review. *Frontiers in Education, 9*, 1206410. https://doi.org/10.3389/feduc.2024.1206410

Park, J. H., Alber-Morgan, S. R., & Cannella-Malone, H. (2011). Effects of mother-implemented picture exchange communication system (PECS) training on independent communicative behaviors of young children with autism spectrum disorders. *Topics in Early Childhood Special Education, 31*(1), 37–47. https://doi.org/10.1177/0271121410393750

Preston, D., & Carter, M. (2009). A review of the efficacy of the picture exchange communication system intervention. *Journal of Autism and Developmental Disorders, 39*(10), 1471–1486. https://doi.org/10.1007/s10803-009-0763-y

Schopler, E., Reichler, R., Bashford, A., Lansing, M., & Marcus, L. (1990). *Individualized assessment and treatment for autistic and developmentally disabled children: Volume 1. Psychoeducational Profile – Revised (PEP-R)*. University Park Press.

Schopler, E., Reichler, R., & Renner, B. (1988). *The childhood autism rating scale (CARS)*. Western Psychological Services.

Schreibman, L., & Stahmer, A. C. (2014). A randomized trial comparison of the effects of verbal and pictorial naturalistic communication strategies on spoken language for young children with autism. *Journal of Autism and Developmental Disorders, 44*(5), 1244–1251. https://doi.org/10.1007/s10803-013-1972-y

Stokes, T. F., & Baer, D. M. (1977). An implicit technology of generalization. *Journal of Applied Behavior Analysis, 10*(2), 349–367. https://doi.org/10.1901/jaba.1977.10-349

van Dijk, W., & Gage, N. A. (2018). The effectiveness of visual activity schedules for individuals with intellectual disabilities: A meta-analysis. *Journal of Intellectual & Developmental Disability, 44*(4), 384–395. https://doi.org/10.3109/13668250.2018.1431761

Chapter 8
Communicating with Speech-Generating Devices

Introduction

At a most basic level, a speech-generating device (SGD) can be defined as any type of technology that produces digitized (i.e., recorded) or synthetic (i.e., computer-generated) speech output. SGDs therefore represent a type of aided communication system. In contrast to other types of aided communication—such as tangible symbols (Chap. 6) and picture exchange (Chap. 7)—SGDs can be seen as representing a more high-tech solution for people with severe disabilities who are nonverbal or minimally verbal. Historically, SGDs were dedicated devices used primarily to replace or augment the limited or unintelligible speech of adults with physical impairments, such as amyotrophic lateral sclerosis or cerebral palsy (Zangari et al., 1994). SGDs have also been used in cases where people have lost their ability to speak due to encephalitis or tracheotomy. Given that many individuals with such conditions tend not to have serious learning impairments, it was likely sufficient to simply show and tell them how to use the device.

Recently, the populations being considered for SGDs—and the popularity of SGDs as an augmentative and alternative communication strategy—have broadened and increased in line with recent technology advances, particularly advances in tablet computers, smartphones, and related portable media devices. These types of devices are multifunctional rather than being dedicated only for use as an SGD. Tablet computers and related types of devices can be configured for use as an SGD by installing any number of increasingly available and affordable speech-generating applications. Such applications typically include a library of communication symbols that produce synthetic speech output when the symbol is selected by the user. For example, Sennott and Bowker (2009) developed an application called Proloquo2Go®, which consists of a large library of icons (i.e., colored line drawings) that produce synthetic speech output when selected. Proloquo2Go® and other such applications enable various mobile devices—such as an iPhone®, iPad®, or

J. Sigafoos et al., *Communication Strategies for People with Severe Disabilities*, Autism and Child Psychopathology Series,
https://doi.org/10.1007/978-3-031-83807-1_8

Apple Watch®[1]—to be used as SGDs. The combination of mobile devices with speech-generating applications does seem to have increased the interest in using SGDs for individuals who are nonverbal, but physically mobile, such as for nonverbal individuals with autism spectrum disorder and/or intellectual disability.

Figure 8.1 shows three SGDs commonly used in communication interventions for nonverbal and minimally verbal people with severe disability. For example, an adolescent with autism might be provided with an iPhone® with the Proloquo2Go® application installed as shown on the left-hand side of Fig. 8.1. Intervention might then focus on teaching the adolescent to tap the icons to communicate various messages. If the person were to tap the *STOP* icon, for example, the device might be programmed to produce some relevant synthesized speech output, such as the phrase, "*Let's take a break.*" To the right of the iPhone device in Fig. 8.1 is a picture of the TD I-110 by Tobii Dynavox®. This is a dedicated touch-screen SGD with preloaded communication software that includes communication symbols and generates naturally sounding speech output. The BIGmack® switch, pictured at the bottom of Fig. 8.1, is a single switch device that can produce up to 2 min of digitized (recorded) speech output. The BIGmack® represents a good choice for individuals at the beginning stages of SGD intervention.

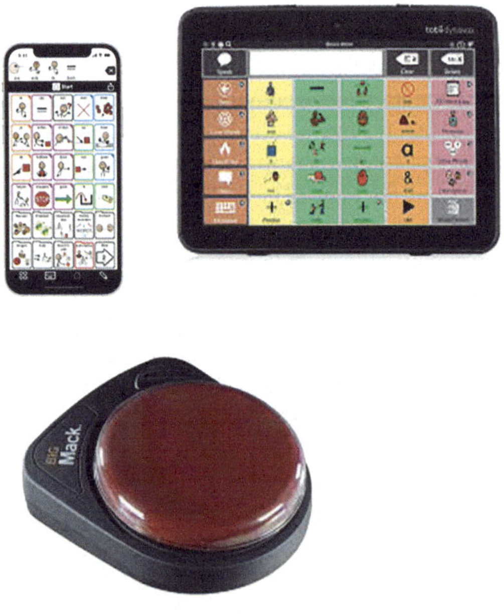

Fig. 8.1 *Examples of SGDs:* Apple iPhone® with the Proloquo2Go®, Tobii Dynavox®, and a BIGmack® switch. *Note:* iPhone® by Apple Inc.; TD I-110 by Tobii Dynavox®, AB (Publ); BIGmack® by AbleNet, Inc.

[1] The iPad®, iPod Touch®, and Apple Watch® are registered trademarks of Apple Inc., 1 Infinite Loop, Cupertino, CA, 95014, USA. www.apple.com. Proloquo2Go® is a registered trademark of AssistiveWare B.V., Laurierstraat 193-1016PL, Amsterdam, The Netherlands.

Systematic Reviews of SGD Intervention Research

Numerous studies have explored the use of SGDs as an alternative or augmentative mode of communication for people with severe disabilities. Indeed, the accumulated research has been synthesized numerous times in systematic reviews. Table 8.1 provides a summary of 10 relevant reviews that have evaluated SGD-based intervention studies. The reviews are grouped by the specific population studied, specifically (a) people with acquired neurological conditions, (b) individuals with autism spectrum disorder, (c) adults with intellectual disability, and (d) individuals with other severe to profound and/or multiple disabilities. Each of these 10 reviews is summarized in terms of number of studies, number and age range of participants, types of SGDs used, and the main findings and/or conclusions arising from the authors' syntheses of the included studies.

Acquired Neurological Conditions

Koul et al. (2010)

This review examined the effectiveness of SGDs as an augmentative communication strategy for people with aphasia. A systematic search identified five studies that used single-case (multiple-baseline) designs and two group design studies. Studies were included if they involved implementation of aided augmentative and alternative communication devices that produced digitized and/or synthetic speech output when a communication symbol or a written text was selected. Additionally, studies had to have measured performance outcomes, such as identifying graphic symbols, responding to questions, describing pictures/videos, and/or producing sentences.

The studies reviewed by Koul et al. (2010) mostly involved participants who were diagnosed with severe aphasia (or Broca's aphasia), characterized by impairments in the production of spontaneous speech and grammatically correct sentences (Acharya & Wroten, 2023). The aims, SGD devices used, procedures, and intervention intensities varied widely across studies, which makes comparisons across studies difficult. In an effort to systematize and quantify the outcomes reported across the five single-case studies, Koul et al. calculated effect sizes for each participant (e.g., each participant's baseline phase compared to their subsequent intervention phase or phases). Effect sizes were classified as indicative of the intervention being either (a) highly effective, (b) fairly effective, (c) questionably effective, or (d) ineffective. About a third of the effect sizes calculated by Koul et al. (i.e., 37%) were considered indicative of a highly effective intervention. In contrast, 17% were classified as fairly effective and the same percentage were deemed to be of questionable effectiveness. The remaining 29% of the effect sizes fell into the ineffective range. Both group studies reviewed by Koul et al. produced effect sizes suggestive of a positive intervention effect. Overall, these calculations reveal a literature

Table 8.1 Summary of 10 systematic reviews evaluating SGD use

Condition/ citation	# of studies	Participants	Types of SGDs	Findings/conclusion
Acquired conditions				
Koul et al. (2010)	7	65 minimally verbal adults (aged 27–86 years) with aphasia	SGDs and computer software with graphic symbols	Results ranged from highly effective to questionably effective
May et al. (2019)	39	573 patients (aged 5–95 years) with dementia	SGDs with digitized or synthetic speech output and nonelectronic/unaided options (e.g., communication books, real objects)	Results were mixed. SGDs appear promising, but require further research
Autism				
van der Meer & Rispoli (2010)	23	51 autistic children (aged 3–16 years)	14 different types of SGDs	Positive results were reported in 86% of the studies
Lorah et al. (2015)	17	57 autistic people (aged 3–23 years)	iPad® or iPod touch® with Proloqu2Go® or related synthetic speech application	93% of participants acquired SGD use
Lorah et al. (2024)	38	106 autistic people (aged 3–44 years)	Six different types of mobile devices, but mainly iPad® and iPod touch®	Positive results were reported for 96% of the participants
Adults with intellectual disability				
Sutherland et al. (2010)	11	15 adults (aged 17–60 years)	9 different types of SGDs	Positive results were reported in 100% of the studies
Boster et al. (2024)	19	43 adults (aged 22–60 years)	13 of the 19 studies evaluated SGDs	Positive results were reported in 100% of the studies
Other severe to profound and multiple disability conditions				
Davis et al. (2010)	14	32 people (aged 1–21 years)	6 of the 19 studies evaluated SGDs	Positive results were reported for 81% of the participants
Rispoli et al. (2010)	35	86 people (aged 1–42 years)	17 different types of SGDs	Positive results were reported in 86% of the studies
Simacek et al. (2018)	25	59 people (aged 2–40 years)	SGDs were used with 24 (40.7%) of the participants	Positive results were reported in 23 (92%) studies and mixed results were reported in 2 studies

characterized by mixed results. This is not surprising given the varied aims, devices, outcome measures, and intervention protocols adopted across studies. In light of this varied literature, Koul et al. made the reasonable conclusion that, while SGDs "seem to be effective," the variability of protocols and the mixed results means that "predictions about the effectiveness of [interventions involving] SGDs for persons with aphasia cannot be made yet" (p. 158).

May et al. (2019)

This review reported on the use of augmentative and alternative communication strategies as a means of supporting memory and expressive and receptive communication in adults with dementia. Both quantitative and qualitative studies involving electronic and nonelectronic devices were included. Their search identified 39 studies, but only 12 of these made use of an electronic communication device. For each included study, the authors summarized a range of variables, including the study's participants, research design, type of communication methods provided, dependent variables, and results.

The cohort of studies reviewed by May et al. (2019) involved a total of 573 patients. These participants were mostly elderly adults with dementia of the Alzheimer's type. Such individuals typically present with impaired memory and thinking processes, in addition to communication difficulty (Jalbert et al., 2008). The interventions procedures employed across these 39 studies varied in terms of intensity and specific procedures, as did the dependent measures and types of communication devices.

Of most relevance to the present chapter are the 12 studies included in the review that made use of electronic communication devices. The specific devices used included iPads® and tablet computers with applications enabling video, audio-recorded sentences, and/or synthetic speech generation via the selection of photographs or other graphic symbols (e.g., an iPad® with the Pictello®[2] application). The 12 studies employing such devices were generally associated with positive outcomes, such as (a) increased vocabulary, (b) reduced utterance ambiguity and repetitions, (c) more on-topic statements, and (d) an overall higher quality and quantity of conversational interactions. However, similar to the Koul et al. (2010) review, the cohort of studies reviewed by May et al. varied considerably in terms of procedures, devices used, outcomes measured, and general methodological quality. This variety is perhaps inevitable in any large cohort of studies, but it does complicate the ability to make comparisons and offer definitive conclusions. In light of this, the main conclusion reached from the May et al. review is that while SGDs appear promising for patients with dementia, further research is required to establish the evidence base necessary to guide clinical practice.

[2] Pictello® is a registered trademark of AssistiveWare B.V., Laurierstraat 193-1016PL, Amsterdam, The Netherlands.

Autism Spectrum Disorder

van der Meer and Rispoli (2010)

This systematic review identified 23 intervention studies that focused on teaching SGD use to children and adolescents with autism. Each of the 23 studies was summarized in terms of its purpose, participants, type of SGDs used, intervention procedures, design, and outcomes. The certainty of evidence provided by each study was also assessed.

The 23 included studies in the van der Meer and Rispoli (2010) review had varying purposes. Most of the studies focused on either (a) evaluating one or more instructional tactics for teaching functional SGD use, (b) comparing acquisition rates and preference for SGDs to other aided and unaided strategies, and/or (c) assessing the role of speech output on participants' production of communication behavior.

In terms of participants, a total of 51 children and adolescents were included across the 23 studies. The children were mainly diagnosed with autism spectrum disorder, although some participants had additional (i.e., intellectual disability, Down syndrome) or related diagnoses (i.e., pervasive developmental disorder not otherwise specified). The 51 children and adolescents ranged from 3 to 16 years of age, with a mean age of 7 years. Most participants were male ($n = 46$ or 90.2%).

A total of 14 different types of SGDs were used across the studies. Most of the SGDs used were of the digitized (i.e., recorded) speech variety (used in 18 or 78% of the studies). Slightly more than half of the studies ($n = 14$ or 61%) provided a rationale for the SGD chosen. The main factors influencing SGD selection related to (a) the participants' motor skills (six studies), (b) the participants' vocabulary needs and/or level of communication ability (five studies), or (c) the specific aims of the study (four studies).

These 23 studies targeted a variety of communication skills, including requesting, social conversation, commenting, answering questions, spelling words, replacing inappropriate speech, and increasing natural speech production. Most studies ($n = 16$ studies or 69.5%) focused on teaching participants to request preferred objects or activities. The next most frequently targeted skills were social conversation and commenting ($n = 6$ or 26% of the studies).

The intervention approaches used in the 23 studies included functional communication training and naturalistic milieu teaching. Generally, the intervention protocols involved (a) creating opportunities by presenting discriminative stimuli or offering preferred items, (b) implementing a constant time-delay procedure (i.e., waiting 10 s for a response to occur), (c) prompting correct responses and correcting errors as necessary, and (d) providing reinforcement. The main types of response prompts used in these studies were graduated guidance, least-to-most prompting, most-to-least prompting, and/or modeling.

In terms of outcomes, 20 studies (87%) were classified as showing a positive intervention effect, meaning that all participants acquired the targeted skills. The remaining three studies (13%) had mixed outcomes, meaning that some but not all participants acquired the targeted skills. All but five studies used single-case experimental designs to evaluate intervention effects and the majority ($n = 18$, 78%) of the studies were rated as providing conclusive evidence of a positive intervention effect. Overall, the studies reviewed by van der Meer and Rispoli (2010) provide good experimental evidence to support the effectiveness of systematic instruction for teaching functional SGD use (i.e., mainly for requesting purposes) to children and adolescents with autism.

Lorah et al. (2015)

Lorah et al. provided a systematic review of intervention studies involving SGDs based on hand-held or tablet computer platforms. They identified 17 studies that evaluated interventions for teaching the use of such devices to individuals with autism and/or related disorders. For each included study, data were extracted on (a) participants' ages and diagnoses, (b) the SGDs used, (c) the communication skills targeted for intervention, (d) the intervention procedures used in teaching the target skills, (e) research design, and (f) outcomes. They also appraised the methodological rigor of the included studies against the 21 quality indicators delineated by Horner et al. (2005). These indicators included (a) operationally defined dependent variables, (b) adequate inter-observer agreement checks, and (c) intervention procedures described in sufficient detail to enable replication.

The 17 studies reviewed by Lorah et al. (2015) included a total of 57 individuals ranging from 3 to 23 years of age. Most participants were preschool or school-aged children. Only one study (van der Meer et al., 2011) included an adult, specifically a 23-year-old woman with severe intellectual disability. (Parenthetically, the 2011 van der Meer et al. study appears to be the first experimental evaluation of an SGD intervention involving a mobile device configured with a commercial speech-generating application. This study's details are summarized in Box 8.1.)

Box 8.1 Summary of the van der Meer et al. (2011) Study

The van der Meer et al. (2011) study appears to be the first empirical study to evaluate the now widely used Proloquo2Go® application. The three participants (Sam, Jim, and Zoe) were 13, 14, and 23 years old, respectively. They all had severe intellectual disability and were either nonverbal (Sam and Zoe) or minimally verbal (Jim). Intervention focused on teaching the participants to request preferred snacks (Sam and Zoe) or preferred snacks and toys (Jim). The SGD was an Apple iPod Touch® with the Proloquo2Go® software application. The device presented a single-screen page containing three icons representing snacks, toys, and social interaction. Tapping each icon activated corresponding synthetic speech output (specifically "*I want a snack please.*", "*Can I play with a toy?*", and *What's new with you?*"). The various phases of the study followed a multiple-probe across participants design to evaluate the effects of intervention. The study began with an initial baseline phase during which the instructor initiated each 5-min session by offering either snacks (Sam and Zoe) or alternating between offers of snacks and toys (Jim) and saying *Let me know if you want snacks (or toys)*. Offers of snacks (or toys) were repeated every 30 s and data were recorded on participants' use of the device, whether the participant reached directly for items, and whether or not the participant consumed/played with a snack/toy that they had obtained by reaching. After baseline, participants received acquisition training. This phase involved implementing a highly structured discrete trial training protocol until participants made three consecutive independent requests for the snacks (Sam and Zoe) or both snacks and toys (Jim). For each trial, the instructor pointed to the available snacks (or toys) and said *Here are some snacks (toys). Let me know if you want something*. For the first three trials, a second instructor, who was positioned behind the participant, immediately used physical guidance to prompt the participant to touch the *SNACK* (or *TOY*) icon. After these first three errorless training trials, a 10-s constant time-delay procedure was programmed before using the physical prompt. Each time the participant made a correct response, whether prompted or not, they received access to the requested snacks (or toys) as natural reinforcement. The social icon was included primarily as a distractor, although tapping it did produce speech output (i.e., "*What's new with you?*"). The toy icon was similarly a distractor for Sam and Zoe. After acquisition training, post-training sessions commenced. During these sessions, various preferred snacks (or toys) were available for 5 min and each correct request was reinforced by allowing the participant to select from the available snacks (or toys). Following the post-training phase, discrimination tests were conducted to rule out possible position-biased and item-biased responding. Follow-up sessions were also conducted with Sam and Jim at 10-week post-training to assess maintenance. The results indicated that the acquisition training procedures were effective in teaching functional use of the SGD to two of the three participants. During baseline, none of the three participants ever used the SGD. When acquisition training was implemented, Sam reached the acquisition criteria for snacks on the ninth training trial. Jim reached acquisition on both snacks and toys on the sixth training trial. During baseline, Zoe began to resist participation. This was seen as her indicating a lack of assent, and therefore she did not continue to participate in the study. Following acquisition, in the post-training phase, both Sam and Jim consistently produced independent requests during each 5-min session. Tests indicated that both boys were making discriminated requests and continued to do so at follow-up. Overall, the results suggest that the use of a discrete trial training protocol involving time delay and physical prompting was effective in promoting subsequent independent and discriminated use of the iPod Touch®-based SGD. This is an important aspect of the study as it suggests there can be rapid acquisition followed by maintenance when the instructional sequence begins with a highly structured and instructor-initiated training paradigm and then shifts to a free-operant (post-training) arrangement, the latter of which is arguably reflective of a more naturalistic communication interaction.

Roughly 75% of the participants in the 17 studies reviewed by Lorah et al. (2015) were listed as having autism spectrum disorder. The remaining participants had other or additional diagnoses, such as intellectual disability, Angelman syndrome, or attention-deficit hyperactivity disorder. In terms of devices, most studies ($n = 11$ or 65%) used an iPod Touch® with the Proloquo2Go® application. The remaining six studies used iPads® with Proloquo2Go® or a comparable application (i.e., GoTalk Now®[3]).

In terms of the communication skills targeted for instruction, 14 or 82% of the studies focused on teaching participants to use their SGDs to make requests. A further two studies taught requesting plus either (a) device operation (e.g., turning on the device, unlocking the screen, and navigating to the application), or (b) social responses, such as greeting the partner, responding to yes/no questions, and using please and thank you. The remaining study targeted commenting or tact responses in response to the questions *What do you see?* and *What is it?*

The intervention procedures implemented for teaching SGD use were mainly some combination of time delay, least-to-most prompting, and reinforcement. These intervention procedures were generally effective in that most participants acquired the targeted SGD-based communication skills relatively quickly. Specifically, across these 17 studies, 93% of the participants (53 out of 57) learned to use the SGD to achieve the targeted communicative skill(s). These positive results support the use of systematic instructional tactics for teaching functional use of iPad®- and iPod Touch®-based SGDs to children and adolescents with autism spectrum disorder and/or related developmental disorders. The evidence reviewed by Lorah et al. can also be viewed as largely conclusive because all of the studies used single-case experimental designs to evaluate the effects of intervention and most (15 of the 17 studies) were also rated as high quality in terms of their overall methodological rigor.

Some interesting comparisons were incorporated into eight of the studies reviewed by Lorah et al. (2015). Specifically, eight studies compared the relative speed of acquisition and/or participants' preference for the SGD versus other communication strategies (e.g., picture exchange and/or manual signing). Five of these eight comparison studies, involving a total of 23 participants, assessed performance with an iPod Touch®- or iPad®-based SGD to both picture exchange and manual signing. In these five studies, 14 of the 23 participants learned to use all three strategies; 6 learned to use two of the three strategies (i.e., SGD and picture exchange); 1 learned to use picture exchange only; and 2 did not reach acquisition with any of the three communication strategies. Two additional studies showed higher rates of requesting for 8 of 10 participants when they used an iPad®-based SGD versus a picture-exchange system. The other two participants performed better with picture exchange. One additional study, involving four participants, compared an iPod Touch® with the Proloqu2Go® application to the use of manual signing. All four

[3]GoTalk Now is a registered trademark of the Attainment Company, Inc., 1158 Clarity Street, Verona, WI 53593-0160, USA.

participants learned to use the SGD to make requests and three of the four also learned to make the same requests with manual signs. Overall, the collective results of these comparison studies indicate that, with intervention, most participants learned to use SGDs, picture exchange, and manual signing. But for some participants, the manual signing intervention was relatively less effective.

In terms of preference, a total of 19 participants from the various comparison studies were provided with structured opportunities to choose whether to use the SGD, picture exchange, or manual signs. In these post-acquisition preference assessments, most participants (16 out of 19) showed a preference for using the SGD, whereas one preferred picture exchange, and the remaining two individuals showed no clear preference. Lorah et al. (2015) speculated that the use of a preferred strategy might increase a person's motivation to communicate. However, the influence of strategy preference on the acquisition, generalization, and/or maintenance of communication skills remains equivocal. Results from numerous studies reviewed in this book (e.g., Chaps. 5, 7, and 8 in particular) indicate that all of the various aided and unaided communication strategies (e.g., manual signs, picture exchange, and SGDs) can be successfully taught and learning often occurs at a comparable rate, although individual differences occur. McLay et al. (2017), for example, taught two nonverbal autistic boys to request more toy play by signing MORE, selecting a laminated *MORE* symbol card, and tapping an icon representing *MORE* from the screen of an iPad®, which then produced synthetic speech output (i.e., "*I want more.*"). Both children showed a clear preference for the SGD, but acquired use of the picture system fastest. Thus, for these two children, preference did not predict the speed of acquisition. Even when differences in acquisition rates emerge, these are often rather modest and thus perhaps clinically irrelevant. Difference in acquisition rates might also indicate that some strategies are simply easier to teach, rather than being inherently easier to learn. In addition, some such differences could reflect varying levels of partner responsivity to the different strategies.

While preference for a particular communication strategy (e.g., SGD versus picture exchange) may not necessarily have a large influence on acquisition, generalization, and/or maintenance, Sigafoos and colleagues (McLay et al.; Sigafoos et al., 2005) argued that enabling participants to indicate their preference is important in its own right and could be one way to incorporate a degree of self-determination into the overall communication intervention process. McLay et al. also suggested that SGDs might be some participants' preferred option because the speech output itself might be reinforcing. In support of this suggestion, McLay et al. cited a study by Sobsey and Reichle (1989). These researchers demonstrated that the auditory output from a call buzzer—which was used to recruit attention—appeared to function as a reinforcer for some of the six individuals with severe disabilities in their study. In contrast, Sigafoos et al. (2003) demonstrated that three nonverbal children—two with autism and one who was blind and had severe intellectual disability—continued to use a BIGmack® switch to request preferred items even when the device was turned off and thus did not produce the recorded speech output ("*I want more*."). That is, requesting occurred at comparable rates whether the recorded message did or did not occur. This suggests that the children were using the SGD functionally to gain access to the preferred items and not simply to hear the noise it made.

Lorah et al. (2024)

A subsequent (2024) review by Lorah et al. sought to document the types of instructional tactics used in teaching autistic individuals to communicate using hand-held devices and tablet-based computers. The review summarized 38 intervention studies, 12 of which had also been included in the previous 2015 review by the same research team. These 38 studies included a total of 106 participants, all of whom had autism spectrum disorder. Participants were predominately male (84%) and ranged from 3 to 44 years of age with a mean age of 7 years and 11 months. A total of six different types of mobile devices and tablet computers were used as SGDs across the 38 studies, but over 80% of the participants were taught to use a speech-generating application—such as Proloquo2Go®—with an iPad® or iPod Touch® device. Consistent with previous reviews, most studies (32 of the 38 studies) targeted mands or requesting behavior. However, many of the studies also targeted additional classes of communicative behavior. The additional communication targets consisted mainly of intraverbal (31 studies) and tacting (25 studies) responses (see Table 5.2 for definitions of mands, tacts, and intraverbals). Also consistent with previous reviews was the finding that structured intervention using systematic instructional tactics (e.g., time delay, response prompting, and reinforcement) was effective. Indeed, with intervention, SGD use increased in all but 4 of the 106 participants. Overall, this review strengthens and extends the evidence base related to the use of iPad®- or iPod Touch®-based SGDs in communication interventions for people with autism spectrum disorders. In particular, the increased variety of communication functions successfully taught represents a significant advance.

Adults with Intellectual Disability

Sutherland et al. (2010)

The question addressed in this review was whether SGDs are a viable communication option for adults with intellectual disability. To address this question, Sutherland et al. identified, summarized, and appraised the evidence from 11 studies that focused on teaching SGD use to adults with intellectual disability. These 11 studies provided intervention to a total of 15 adults (aged 18–60 years). This cohort of 15 adults included nonverbal and minimally verbal people and roughly equal numbers had severe/profound versus moderate/mild intellectual disability. Nine different types of SGDs were used including switches linked to tape recorders and dedicated devices, such as the TouchTalker® with Minispeak®[4] symbols.

A variety of communicative skills, interactions, or functions were targeted for intervention across the 11 studies. Five studies taught participants to use SGDs to make various types of requests, specifically requesting access to preferred objects (three studies), requesting information (one study), and placing an order at a fast-food restaurant (one study). The other studies focused on teaching SGD use for social interactions, task-related communication, to ask and answer questions, and/or general sentence production.

The intervention approaches used in most studies (7 of the 11 studies and 11 of the 15 adult participants) involved the application of some combination of various systematic instructional tactics, such as (a) presenting a discriminative stimulus to create a teaching opportunity, (b) prompting SGD use, and (c) reinforcement. Overall, all of the participants reportedly learned to use their respective SGDs for the targeted communication purpose(s). However, only 4 of the 11 studies were rated as being capable of providing conclusive evidence. In the remaining seven studies, the evidence was rated as inconclusive due to reliance on pre-experimental designs, limited procedural descriptions, and/or insufficient reliability data. Thus, the amount and quality of evidence provided in the 11 studies reviewed by Sutherland et al. is limited in terms of methodological quality, but evidence from the four higher quality studies suggest that SGDs can be successfully taught to, and may therefore represent a viable communication strategy for nonverbal and minimally verbal adults with intellectual disability.

Boster et al. (2024)

In light of the limited amount of high-quality evidence noted by Sutherland et al. (2010), the more recent 2024 review by Boster et al. represents a timely and much-needed update of the literature. This research team identified 19 studies that were published over a span of 28 years (1992–2020).[5] These 19 studies provided SGD intervention to 43 adults ranging from 22 to 60 years of age and with a mean age of 38 years. Participants mainly had moderate-to-severe intellectual disability along with more specific diagnoses (e.g., cerebral palsy or Down syndrome). Of the 19 studies, 6 used various high-tech communication strategies and another 7 incorporated the use of both high-tech and lower-tech aided systems. Unfortunately, the authors did not define the term high-tech nor specify the exact types of high-tech

[4]Touch Talker® with Minspeak®, Prentke Romich Company (PRC), 1022 Heyl Road, Wooster, OH 44691, USA. This device became available in 1984 and was, at that time, one of the few portable SGDs.

[5]The number of studies identified by Boster et al. (2024) is relatively low compared to the number and recency of studies involving children with autism spectrum disorder. This suggests that adults with intellectual disability might be underserved and under-represented in the SGD literature.

devices used. Still, it is likely that their definition of high-tech covered SGDs because there are references to voice output communication aids and speech output.

Boster et al. (2024) classified target skills as social, linguistic, operational, or strategic. Social skills (e.g., initiating, maintaining, and terminating social interactions) were targeted in 11 studies. Linguistic skills (e.g., expressive and receptive language and knowledge of the linguistic code) were targeted in nine studies. Operational skills (i.e., the technical skills required to operate the device) were targeted in six studies. And one study aimed to develop strategic skills, which were defined as "Compensatory strategies used to deal with functional limitations associated with AAC" (p. 2).

In terms of outcomes, most studies (14 out of the 19 studies involving 32 of the 43 adult participants) reported positive results. The other five studies reported mixed results. About half of the studies (n = 9) had methodological concerns, which reduces the certainty of evidence, Boster et al. (2024) concluded there is a benefit to the use of aided communication strategies in communication interventions for adults with intellectual disability. These reviewers also noted the importance of training communicative partners to be responsive to the adult's use of an SGD. Responsiveness includes implementing evidence-based strategies—such as milieu teaching—to facilitate the use of the aided communication device by the adult with intellectual disability.

Other Severe to Profound and Multiple Disability Conditions

Davis et al. (2010)

In this review, 14 intervention studies were found that focused on teaching expressive use of aided communication strategies to people with hearing impairment and additional intellectual, developmental, and/or physical disabilities. This is an important population focus given that hearing impairment is prevalent among people with intellectual and other developmental disabilities (Danyluk & Jacob, 2023).

Of the 14 studies identified by Davis et al. (2010), 6 focused on teaching SGD use, the other studies taught low-tech strategies (e.g., communication boards). The six SGD studies provided intervention to a total of nine participants, all but one of whom were children from 2 to 8 years of age. The other participant was a 20-year-old female. In terms of target skills, two participants were taught to use an SGD to request preferred stimuli. One participant was taught to recruit attention using an SGD. Another study, with two participants, taught commenting skills. The remaining two studies, with a total of four participants, targeted multiple communication skills (e.g., recruiting attention, requesting preferred stimuli, and/or commenting).

Most of the intervention packages implemented consisted of some combination of systematic instructional procedures, such as least-to-most prompting, most-to-least prompting, graduated guidance, and/or time delay, as well as reinforcement. Davis et al. (2010) classified each study's outcomes in terms of whether improvement in the targeted skills was evident for (a) all participants in the study, (b) some participants in the study, or (c) none of the study's participants. By these criteria, six participants from five of the six studies using SGDs "demonstrated evident improvement." Mixed results were reported in one study, indicating that some but not all of the three participants in that study showed acquisition of the targeted skills. Overall, while the evidence base is sparse, the results of this review suggest that SGDs could represent a viable communication strategy for some people with developmental disability and hearing impairment. While many such individuals would likely be "unable to hear the auditory output" (Davis et al., p. 253) from the SGD, that output could still be quite useful to communication partners.

Rispoli et al. (2010)

This review summarized 35 SGD-based intervention studies involving people with cerebral palsy, intellectual disability, and/or multiple disabilities. In these 35 studies, intervention to establish functional SGD use was provided to a total of 86 participants. Participants ranged from 1 to 42 years of age, with a mean age of 12.9 years. Most (70%) participants were diagnosed with intellectual disability. Other diagnoses included Angelman syndrome, cerebral palsy, Down syndrome, and spina bifida. Fifty-five percent of the sample ($n = 47$ participants) were described as having multiple disabilities. Most participants were classified as either nonverbal ($n = 60$ or 70%) or as having fewer than 10 spoken words ($n = 25$ or 29%). Most participants were taught to use an SGD to make requests (58%), followed by (a) social etiquette (e.g., "*Thank you*") responses (27%), (b) using appropriate syntax (7%), (c) labeling (4%), and (d) answering questions (2%). Relatively few participants (i.e., 2%) were taught more than one communication skill.

Seventeen different types of SGDs were used across the 35 studies reviewed by Rispoli et al. (2010). Single switch devices, which allowed for only a single communicative message to be produced, were used with 46% of the participants. SGDs with greater message capacity (i.e., anywhere from 2–37+ symbol/message options) were used with the remaining participants. Interventions were classified as either involving discrete trial training, milieu teaching, or a combination of approaches. Discrete trial training, which was used in 26 of the 35 studies, involved (a) clearly presenting discriminative stimuli to initiate teaching opportunities, (b) response prompting and error correction, and (c) contingent reinforcement of correct responses. Milieu teaching approaches, which were used in seven studies, involved (a) following the participant's lead, (b) incorporating teaching opportunities into natural routines, (c) response prompting, and (d) natural reinforcement. The final two studies combined aspects of both discrete trial training and milieu teaching approaches.

In terms of outcomes, each of the 35 studies was classified as providing (a) positive, (b) mixed, or (c) negative outcomes depending on whether target skills improved for (a) all participants, (b) some, but not all participants, or (c) for none of the participants. Most studies ($n = 30$ or 86%) reported positive outcomes. The remaining studies reported mixed outcomes. Given that all but four studies used experimental designs and a majority of the studies (54%) were deemed capable of providing conclusive evidence, the overall results of this review suggest that discrete trial training and milieu teaching can be successfully applied to enable SGD-based communication in nonverbal and minimally verbal people with a range of developmental and physical/multiple disabilities.

Simacek et al. (2018)

This research team systematically searched for intervention studies focused on teaching aided communication strategies to people with severe to profound and multiple disabilities. Their search uncovered 25 studies that (a) used a single-case experimental design, (b) involved the provision of an intervention aimed at increasing one or more communication behaviors, and (c) included at least one participant who was nonverbal or minimally verbal (i.e., five or fewer spoken words) due to a severe or profound level of intellectual/developmental disability and/or multiple (e.g., intellectual and sensory and/or physical) disabilities. Interventions involving various types of aided strategies were considered, specifically microswitch technology, two-dimensional picture-based strategies, three-dimensional tangible symbols, and SGDs.

The 25 studies included a total of 59 participants (31 females and 28 males) ranging from 2 to 40 years of age, with the majority of participants (74.6%) being school-aged children (aged 6–18 years). A variety of diagnoses were represented among the 59 participants including Rett syndrome (13.6%), cerebral palsy (10.2%), autism (10.2%), Angelman syndrome (5.1%), and Down syndrome (1.7%). More than half the sample (59.3%) were blind or visually impaired and 11.9% had hearing impairment. Almost half of the participants ($n = 24$ or 40.7%) were taught to use an SGD, mostly for requesting purposes (e.g., requesting preferred stimuli and/or requesting attention). The teaching procedures mainly involved the use of systematic instructional tactics (e.g., time delay, verbal cueing, least-to-most prompting, modeling, and reinforcement).

An important set of variables considered in this review related to intervention intensity or dosage. Specifically, where available, Simacek et al. (2018) recorded the number and length of intervention sessions as well as the number of teaching opportunities provided within the sessions. A fairly typical arrangement—found in roughly half the studies—had participants receiving four, 10-min sessions per week over a 3–4-month period and with each session incorporating about six (or more) teaching opportunities. This equates to about 8–10 total intervention hours and roughly 288–385 total teaching opportunities.

Overall, these figures suggest that many of the intervention protocols applied were of relatively modest intensity. However, it is important to note these dosages were sufficient to achieve positive outcomes. In fact, all of the SGD studies reviewed by Simacek et al. (2018) indicated gains for either all or most participants. And because these studies employed rigorous experimental designs (e.g., multiple baseline, multiple probe, ABAB/withdrawal, and adapted alternating treatments designs), the resulting data provide convincing evidence that the positive effects were most likely due to the implementation of the intervention procedures. In summary, the Simacek et al. review supports the use of systematic instructional procedures for teaching functional SGD use to people with various types of severe to profound and multiple disabilities.

Indications for Use of SGDs

Based on results from the 10 systematic reviews summarized in Table 8.1, SGDs can be indicated for a range of neurological and developmental disorders that compromise natural speech production and/or spoken language acquisition. SGDs may be indicated when there is a need to provide an alternative (nonspeech) communication strategy for people who are unlikely to acquire speech. SGDs are also indicated for augmenting limited or unintelligible speech. More generally, SGDs are intended to enable communication when speech is either temporarily or permanently insufficient to meet the person's everyday communication needs.

Researchers have highlighted a number of potential advantages associated with SGDs. Wendt et al. (2019), for example, noted that the auditory/speech output from an SGD may be easy for communication partners to understand because of its similarity to natural speech. However, the ease with which SGD output can be interpreted by communication partners may depend on a number of variables. As delineated by Drager et al. (2010), these variables include the (a) intelligibility or acoustical quality of the speech output, (b) the rate at which the output occurs, (c) contextual cues surrounding the communicative exchange, (d) partners' familiarity with the SGD user and previous experience with SGD output, and (e) partners' level of receptive language ability.

Like natural speech, use of an SGD has a built-in or automatic attention-recruitment aspect to it. This is an advantage because the communication partner does not necessarily have to be present and attending to the person in order for the intended message to be successfully transmitted (Sobsey & Reichle, 1989). Furthermore, many SGDs can be programmed to produce messages so detailed (e.g., "*I would like an Americano with a splash of oat milk.*") that the potential for misunderstanding is minimized.

Another potential advantage noted by Wendt et al. (2019) is that the speech output from an SGD might represent a type of modeling prompt that could in turn facilitate the user's natural speech production. Several studies provide some support for this suggestion. Roche et al. (2014), for example, taught two minimally verbal boys with neurodevelopmental disorders to use an iPad®-based SGD to request preferred stimuli. These researchers observed that both boys began to utter relevant single words during SGD intervention. In another relevant study, Gervarter et al. (2016) provided an SGD-based communication intervention to four minimally verbal autistic boys and found that three of the four participants "began emitting vocal word approximations with SGD responses" (p. 17). However, these word approximations occurred only "after vocal instructional methods (delays, differential reinforcement, prompting) were introduced" (p. 17). The results suggest that the addition of speech-based instruction to an SGD intervention may increase vocal output in some children. In a systematic replication of the Gevarter et al. study, Bishop et al. (2020) found a similarly facilitative effect for three autistic children when imitative/echoic prompting was added to the SGD-based intervention. These results suggest that there could be ways to deliver an SGD intervention that "may lead to increased vocal output for children with autism spectrum disorder" (Bishop et al., 2020, p. 475).

Contraindications to the Use of SGDs

Historically, as mentioned earlier in this chapter, SGDs were primarily used with nonambulatory people and the device was affixed to their wheelchair. Thus, portability was not a major consideration. With ambulatory people, however, portability needs to be considered. It can be problematic to use an SGD that is not within easy reach because it must first be located/retrieved and powered-up/turned on. The person must then navigate to the screen page holding the required communication symbols and select the correct symbols with sufficient fineness to activate the corresponding speech output. The need to complete a sequence of steps may slow the speed of communication, disrupt conversational turn-taking, limit spontaneity, and perhaps even prevent the person from being able to communicate when the device is out of reach or otherwise unavailable (e.g., due to the need for recharging or a software update). However, just as the use of SGD for communicating requests, comments, and other messages has been successfully taught using systematic instructional procedures, so too have the various operational aspects of SGD use been taught. Sigafoos et al. (2004), for example, used time delay and least-to-most prompting to teach three nonverbal participants with developmental disabilities to search for and retrieve their SGD when it was placed out of reach in various classroom locations. People with severe disabilities have also been taught to power-up and unlock their SGDs screens and navigate to the correct screen page using time delay, least-to-most prompting, and reinforcement (Achmadi et al., 2012).

Another potential barrier to SGD use relates to the fact that many such devices (e.g., an iPhone® or iPad®) require precise motor skills to operate, such as lightly tapping screen icons and swiping left and right to navigate between screens (Wendt et al., 2019). Again, systematic instruction may be helpful for teaching these types of operational skills. Kagohara et al. (2010), for example, worked with an adolescent with autism who initially failed to successfully activate the speech output when using an iPod Touch® as an SGD. Specifically, this person initially tried to work the device by pressing, rather than lightly tapping, his communication symbols. To overcome this problem, the researchers shaped up a more effective tapping response using time delay, response prompting, and differential reinforcement.

Given that these types of operational skills can be taught, the initial lack of such skills should not necessarily contraindicate a person's candidacy for SGD intervention. On the other hand, Wendt et al. (2019) pointed out that certain motor, cognitive, and/or sensory impairments will likely compromise a person's ability to gain independence with certain types of SGDs. For example, SGDs that require the user to directly select icons from small visual displays—such as is required with an iPhone®—would likely be contraindicated for blind people and those lacking fine motor control. For people who are not able to directly select communication symbols on SGD due to motor control problems, various assistive technology solutions could be considered (see Chap. 9).

Cost is another factor that may impact decisions related to selecting SGDs. Because SGDs are more expensive than the other communication strategies covered in this book, their use might be difficult to justify in the absence of evidence that the person would prefer such a device and could be taught to care for it and use it functionally.

As mentioned previously, it is possible that some individuals might come to use SGDs simply to produce the noise those devices make rather than to communicate specific messages to a partner. The former situation would be evidenced if the person repeatedly activated the device even when there were no communication partners present or if the person continued to activate the device even when a communication partner had responded to the presumed intent of the person's communicative act. Such evidence may not necessarily contraindicate SGD intervention, but may rather signal the need to modify intervention to ensure the SGD comes to be used as a tool for communication, rather than merely as an expensive noise-making toy. Ensuring functional use of an SGD for communication purposes is perhaps more likely to occur when use of the device leads to social or tangible outcomes that are more reinforcing than the auditory (speech output) simulation.

Implementation Considerations

Davis et al. (2010) noted that SGD intervention "requires considerations above and beyond those" for other aided strategies (p. 249). These considerations include the need for either the user and/or communication partners (e.g., parents, peers, siblings, teachers, and speech-language pathologists) to have competencies related to maintaining and programming the device. With respect to maintenance, Shepherd et al. (2009) found some reasons to question the reliability of SGDs. Their survey data indicated that such devices often failed within the first 42 weeks of use. In addition, 40% required some type of repair within the first year. Failures and the need for repair were mostly due to problems with touch screens, wiring, batteries, memory cards, and charging issues. In terms of programming SGDs, this often requires a number of steps, including selecting vocabulary/communication symbols and loading or recording the corresponding speech output for each communication icon or symbol. Programming considerations also include how to arrange the symbols, such as in a grid or by embedding hotspots within a photographic scene. Symbols should be arranged in a way that will best facilitate the user's ease of communicating. Wilkinson et al. (2012) suggest that individual differences in visual-cognitive processing may impact a person's use of symbol displays, such as a visual scene display. Gevarter et al. (2014) found individual differences among three autistic children. Two of the three children learned to make SGD-based requests faster when their communication symbols consisted of photographs that more closely resembled the size and location of the corresponding real object compared to a line drawing presentation. The other child performed comparably on both formats.

Another consideration is whether to use static or animated communication symbols. Animating communication symbols—to either cue/prompt correct responses or to provide feedback for correct responses—is now a relatively easy programming option. In a review of the literature on the use of animated communication symbols, Schlosser et al. (2022) concluded that animating symbols may facilitate symbol recognition and understanding for some individuals.

A further consideration is the type of SGD. There are many different types of SGDs, and the type of device best suited to any given individuals is likely to change over time as the person's communication competencies and needs evolve. Reichle and colleagues described a process of modality sampling in which a person's performance with different communication strategies is directly compared (Martin et al., 2013; Reichle et al., 1991). This approach could be used to identify which of several different types of SGDs might be best suited to any given individual. Specifically, the person's performance with, and preference for, several different SGDs could be directly compared during a structured intervention trial. Overall, the selection of an SGD—and the selection and display of communication symbols for use with an SGD—is an important consideration that is perhaps best made at the individual level.

Summary and Conclusion

SGDs that produce digitized (i.e., recorded) or synthetic (i.e., computer-generated) speech output are increasingly being used as an aided augmentative and alternative communication strategy for nonverbal and minimally verbal people with severe disabilities. Numerous studies have demonstrated effective procedures for teaching SGD use to individuals with a range of disability conditions. The evidence base is particularly strong for children with autism spectrum disorder. There have also been a fairly good number of studies demonstrating successful SGD use by adults with intellectual disability, as well as individuals with severe to profound and multiple disabilities. Some positive results have also been reported for patients with aphasia and dementia. Individuals with these types of disability conditions have been successfully taught to use SGDs to accomplish a number of specific communication functions; mostly requesting, but also labeling, commenting, answering questions, academic takes (e.g., producing sentences), and social communication (e.g., greeting others and initiating conversation).

Wendt et al. (2019) noted that there is no standard or single protocol for SGD interventions. However, the literature summarized in Table 8.1 indicates that functional use of SGDs has been successfully taught using the same type of systematic instructional procedures that have been proven to be consistently effective in teaching and enhancing peoples' use of the other communication strategies considered in this book (e.g., prelinguistic behaviors, natural gestures, manual signs, tangible symbols, and picture exchange). Indeed, based on the evidence reviewed in this chapter, successful SGD intervention may depend largely on the quality of instruction. While it may be sufficient for some people to simply provide them with an SGD and tell and show them how to use it, other people will likely require more systematic, structured, and explicit instruction.

The speech output from SGDs is a potential advantage that may facilitate communication. Cost and portability are potential disadvantages. The person's preferences, motor skills, and visual-cognitive processing abilities are factors to consider when designing an SGD intervention. In conclusion, data support SGDs as a viable communication strategy for people with a range of neurological and developmental disorders that compromise natural speech production and/or spoken language acquisition.

References

Acharya, A. B., & Wroten, M. (2023). Broca aphasia. https://www.ncbi.nlm.nih.gov/books/NBK436010/

Achmadi, D., Kagohara, D. M., van der Meer, L., O'Reilly, M. F., Lancioni, G. E., Sutherland, D., Lang, R., Marschik, P. B., Green, V. A., & Sigafoos, J. (2012). Teaching advanced operation of an iPad-based speech-generating device to two students with autism spectrum disorders. *Research in Autism Spectrum Disorders, 6*(4), 1258–1264. https://doi.org/10.1016/j.rasd.2012.05.005

Bishop, S. K., Moore, J. W., Dart, E. H., Radley, K., Brewer, R., Barker, L. K., Quintero, L., Litten, S., Gilfeather, A., Newborne, B., & Toche, C. (2020). Further investigation of increasing vocalizations of children with autism with a speech-generating device. *Journal of Applied Behavior Analysis, 53*(1), 475–483. https://doi.org/10.1002/jaba.554

Boster, J. B., Miller Sonntag, A., Evans, A., & Lou, A. (2024). Aided augmentative and alternative communication intervention for adults with developmental disabilities: A scoping review. *International Journal of Developmental Disabilities*. https://doi.org/10.1080/20473869.2024.2366725

Danyluk, A., & Jacob, R. (2023). Hearing loss diagnosis and management in adults with intellectual and developmental disabilities. *Advances in Medicine, 2023*, 6825476. https://doi.org/10.1155/2023/6825476

Davis, T. N., Barnard-Brak, L., Dacus, S., & Pond, A. (2010). Aided AAC systems among individuals with hearing loss and disabilities. *Journal of Developmental and Physical Disabilities, 22*(3), 241–256. https://doi.org/10.1007/s10882-009-9180-6

Drager, K., Reichle, J., & Pinkowski, C. (2010). Synthesized speech output and children: A scoping review. *American Journal of Speech-Language Pathology, 19*(3), 259–273. https://doi.org/10.1044/1058-0360(2010/09-0024)

Gervarter, C., O'Reilly, M. F., Kuhn, M., Mills, K., Ferguson, R., Watkins, L., Sigafoos, J., Lang, R., Rojeski, L., & Lancioni, G. E. (2016). Increasing the vocalizations of individuals with autism during intervention with a speech-generating device. *Journal of Applied Behavior Analysis, 49*(1), 17–33. https://doi.org/10.1002/jaba.270

Gevarter, C., O'Reilly, M. F., Rojeski, L., Sammarco, N., Sigafoos, J., Lancioni, G., & Lang, R. (2014). Comparing acquisition of AAC-based mands in three young children with autism spectrum disorder using iPad® applications with different display and design elements. *Journal of Autism and Developmental Disorders, 44*(10), 2464–2474. https://doi.org/10.1007/s10803-014-2115-9

Horner, R. H., Carr, E. G., Halle, J., McGee, G., Odom, S., & Wolery, M. (2005). The use of single-subject research to identify evidence-based practice in special education. *Exceptional Children, 71*(2), 165–179. https://doi.org/10.1177/001440290507100203

Jalbert, J. J., Daiello, L. A., & Lapane, K. L. (2008). Dementia of the Alzheimer type. *Epidemiologic Reviews, 30*(1), 15–34. https://doi.org/10.1093/epirev/mxn008

Kagohara, D. M., van der Meer, L., Achmadi, D., Green, V. A., O'Reilly, M. F., Mulloy, A., Lancioni, G. E., Lang, R., & Sigafoos, J. (2010). Behavioral intervention promotes successful use of an iPod-based communication device by an adolescent with autism. *Clinical Case Studies, 9*(5), 328–338. https://doi.org/10.1177/1534650110379633

Koul, R., Petroi, D., & Schosser, R. W. (2010). Systematic review of speech generating devices for aphasia. In J. Mullennix & S. Stern (Eds.), *Computer synthesized speech technologies: Tools for aiding impairment* (pp. 148–160). IGI Global.

Lorah, E. R., Holyfield, C., Griffen, B., & Caldwell, N. (2024). A systematic review of evidence-based instruction for individuals with autism using mobile augmentative and alternative communication technology. *Review Journal of Autism and Developmental Disorders, 11*(1), 210–224. https://doi.org/10.1007/s40489-022-00334-6

Lorah, E. R., Parnell, A., Schaefer Whitby, P., & Hantula, D. (2015). A systematic review of tablet computers and portable media players as speech generating devices for individuals with autism spectrum disorder. *Journal of Autism and Developmental Disorders, 45*(12), 3792–3804. https://doi.org/10.1007/s10803-014-2314-4

Martin, J. H., Reichle, J., Dimian, A., & Chen, M. (2013). Communication modality sampling for a toddler with Angelman syndrome. *Language, Speech, and Hearing Services in Schools, 44*(4), 327–336. https://doi.org/10.1044/0161-1461(2013/12-0108)

May, A. A., Dada, S., & Murray, J. (2019). Review of AAC interventions for persons with dementia. *International Journal of Language and Communication Disorders, 54*(6), 857–874. https://doi.org/10.1111/1460-6984.12491

McLay, L., Schafer, M., van der Meer, L., Couper, L., McKenzie, E., O'Reilly, M. F., Lancioni, G. E., Marschik, P. B., Sigafoos, J., & Sutherland, D. (2017). Acquisition, preference and follow-up comparison across three AAC modalities taught to two children with autism spectrum disorder. *International Journal of Disability, Development and Education, 64*(2), 117–130. https://doi.org/10.1080/1034912X.2016.1188892

Reichle, J., York, J., & Sigafoos, J. (1991). *Implementing augmentative and alternative communication: Strategies for learners with severe disabilities*. Paul H. Brookes Publishing Co.

Rispoli, M. J., Franco, J. H., van der Meer, L., Lang, R., & Camargo, S. P. (2010). The use of speech generating devices in communication interventions for individuals with developmental disabilities: A review of the literature. *Developmental Neurorehabilitation, 13*(4), 276–293. https://doi.org/10.3109/17518421003636794

Roche, L., Sigafoos, J., Lancioni, G. E., O'Reilly, M. F., Schlosser, R. W., Stevens, M., van der Meer, L., Achmadi, D., Kagohara, D., James, R., Carnett, A., Hodis, F., Green, V. A., Sutherland, D., Lang, R., Rispoli, M., Machalicek, W., & Marschik, P. B. (2014). An evaluation of speech production in two boys with neurodevelopmental disorders who received communication intervention with a speech-generating device. *International Journal of Developmental Neuroscience, 38*(1), 10–16. https://doi.org/10.1016/j.ijdevneu.2014.07.003

Schlosser, R. W., Choe, N., Koul, R., Shane, H. C., Yu, C., & Wu, M. (2022). Roles of animation in augmentative and alternative communication: A scoping review. *Current Developmental Disorders Reports, 9*(4), 187–203. https://doi.org/10.1007/s40474-022-00255-3

Sennott, S., & Bowker, A. (2009). Autism, AAC, and Proloquo2Go. *Perspectives on Augmentative and Alternative Communication, 18*(4), 137–145. https://doi.org/10.1044/aac18.4.137

Shepherd, T. A., Campbell, K. A., Renzoni, A. M., & Sloan, N. (2009). Reliability of speech generating devices: A 5-year review. *Augmentative and Alternative Communication, 25*(3), 145–153. https://doi.org/10.1080/07434610902996104

Sigafoos, J., Didden, R., & O'Reilly, M. (2003). Effects of speech output on the maintenance of requesting and frequency of vocalizations in three children with developmental disabilities. *Augmentative and Alternative Communication, 19*(1), 37–47. https://doi.org/10.1080/0743461032000056487

Sigafoos, J., O'Reilly, M., Ganz, J., Lancioni, G., & Schlosser, R. (2005). Supporting self-determination in AAC interventions by assessing preference for communication devices. *Technology & Disability, 17*(3), 143–153.

Sigafoos, J., O'Reilly, M., Seely-York, S., & Edrisinha, C. (2004). Teaching students with developmental disabilities to locate their AAC device. *Research in Developmental Disabilities, 25*(4), 371–383. https://doi.org/10.1016/j.ridd.2003.07002

Simacek, J., Pennington, B., Reichle, J., & Parker-McGowan, Q. (2018). Aided AAC for people with severe to profound and multiple disabilities: A systematic review of interventions and treatment intensity. *Advances in Neurodevelopmental Disorders, 2*(1), 100–115. https://doi.org/10.1007/s41252-017-0050-4

Sobsey, D., & Reichle, J. (1989). Components of reinforcement for attention signal switch activation. *Mental Retardation & Learning Disability Bulletin, 17*(2), 46–59.

Sutherland, D., Sigafoos, J., Schlosser, R. W., O'Reilly, M. F., & Lancioni, G. E. (2010). Are speech-generating devices viable AAC options for adults with intellectual disabilities? In J. Mullennix & S. Stern (Eds.), *Computer synthesized speech technologies: Tools for aiding impairment* (pp. 161–176). IGI Global.

van der Meer, L., Kagohara, D., Achmadi, D., Green, V. A., Herrington, C., Sigafoos, J., O'Reilly, M. F., Lancioni, G. E., Lang, R., & Rispoli, M. (2011). Teaching functional use of an iPod-based speech-generating device to individuals with developmental disabilities. *Journal of Special Education Technology, 26*(3), 1–11. https://doi.org/10.1177/016264341102600301

van der Meer, L., & Rispoli, M. (2010). Communication interventions involving speech-generating devices for children with autism: A review of the literature. *Developmental Neurorehabilitation, 13*(4), 294–306. https://doi.org/10.3109/17518421003671494

Wendt, O., Hsu, N., Simon, K., Dienhart, A., & Cain, L. (2019). Effects of an iPad-based speech-generating device infused into instruction with the picture exchange communication system for adolescents and young adults with severe autism spectrum disorder. *Behavior Modification, 43*(6), 898–932. https://doi.org/10.1177/0145445519870552

Wilkinson, K. M., Light, J., & Drager, K. (2012). Considerations for the composition of visual scene displays: Potential contributions of information from visual and cognitive sciences. *Augmentative and Alternative Communication, 28*(3), 137–147. https://doi.org/10.3109/07434618.2012.704522

Zangari, C., Lloyd, L., & Vicker, B. (1994). Augmentative and alternative communication: An historic perspective. *Augmentative and Alternative Communication, 10*(1), 27–59. https://doi.org/10.1080/07434619412331276740

Chapter 9
Assistive Technology Solutions for Enabling People with Intellectual and Motor or Sensory-Motor Disabilities to Access Communication Events

Introduction

People with combinations of intellectual, motor, and sensory impairments face numerous challenges in critical areas of their daily life (e.g., areas concerning functional occupation, access to leisure events, and communication) (Badia et al., 2013; Desideri et al., 2021; Dijkhuizen et al., 2016; Lancioni et al., 2023a; Maes et al. 2021, Nijs & Maes 2021). For example, they (a) may have limited contact with their surroundings and a tendency to be passive and detached, (b) may be unable to operate conventional devices, such as television and computers, that are instrumental for activating leisure events, and (c) may lack verbal skills and also present with serious or extreme limitations in using nonverbal communication means (Chan et al., 2013; Danker et al., 2023; Darcy et al., 2017; Desideri et al., 2021; Ricci et al., 2017). Given the importance of improving their situation, intervention programs have been developed within each of the aforementioned areas. For example, efforts to provide people extra opportunities to access leisure (pleasant) events have led to the development of programs characterized by environmental enrichment, use of multisensory rooms or multisensory storytelling, and introduction of microswitch-based technology ensuring the delivery of stimulation contingent on some forms of functional/adaptive behavior (Kotloski & Sutula, 2015; Lancioni et al., 2024c; Munde & Vlaskamp, 2015; Rushton et al., 2023; Ten Brug et al., 2016).

Efforts to support people's occupation and physical activity have led to the development of programs characterized by the use of exercise devices designed to (a) guide people's activation and movement (e.g., assisted pedaling) or (b) motivate them to perform specific movements through the use of interactive technology, that

J. Sigafoos et al., *Communication Strategies for People with Severe Disabilities*, Autism and Child Psychopathology Series,
https://doi.org/10.1007/978-3-031-83807-1_9

is, technology ensuring the delivery of movement-contingent stimulation (Burns et al., 2022; Hassan et al., 2019; Lancioni et al., 2024a). Efforts to promote people's communication have prompted the development of a variety of intervention programs characterized by different goals and relying on different means, programs that have been presented and analyzed in other chapters of this book.

The scope of the present chapter is to extend the analysis of the options available for helping people with disabilities in the communication area. In particular, the chapter focuses on the presentation and analysis of intervention programs and supporting technology solutions that make communication events accessible to people with intellectual, motor, or sensory-motor disabilities (i.e., people for whom most of the strategies discussed in the other chapters of this book could be largely unsuitable). The first three sections of the chapter focus on programs directed at helping people with severe/profound intellectual disability (or cognitive disability following traumatic brain injury) combined with extensive motor or sensory-motor impairments. These participants tend to remain passive and have no real effective means to interact with their context and make requests (Lancioni et al., 2024c, Roche et al., 2015). Moreover, they do not seem to be able to use communication strategies not supported by assistive technology (e.g., manual signs and pictorial exchange communication systems) or common technology-aided strategies available in this area (e.g., speech-generating devices) (Lancioni et al., 2024d).

The fourth section of the chapter focuses on programs for people who have moderate levels of intellectual disability, are capable and willing to interact with their context, are interested in different forms of environmental stimulation and/or different types of activities, and thus would be expected to make multiple requests to access all those events that they find interesting. The problem with them is that they may not be able to use the communication systems available for making those requests due to serious sensory or sensory-motor impairments (Lancioni et al., 2023b, 2024a). The development of new interventions with new forms of technology can provide these people with the means necessary to express themselves (i.e., to make their requests in a way that is immediately clear to staff and caregivers).

The fifth section of the chapter focuses on programs that might help people with moderate intellectual disability and motor or sensory-motor impairments (a) engage in a different form of communication compared to those pursued by the previous programs (i.e., in interacting with distant partners rather than in making requests) and (b) also get involved in leisure activities and functional tasks (Lancioni et al., 2020, 2023a). The final three sections of the chapter analyze (a) the conditions necessary to make the programs and related technology solutions applicable and effective, (b) the level of accessibility and practicality of the programs, and (c) the question of whether the programs are temporary or long-term solutions.

Section 1: Programs Involving the Use of Microswitches to Allow People with Severe/Profound Intellectual and Sensory-Motor Disabilities to Request/Access Environmental Stimulation

A large number of people with severe/profound intellectual and extensive sensory-motor disabilities may not manage to establish direct connection with their context (e.g., objects and stimulation) and need some form of technology support (e.g., the use of one or more microswitches) to do so. Microswitches are simple devices that can be activated via a variety of small movements and thus are also suitable for participants with severe or extensive motor impairments. They are typically linked to a computer, tablet, or smartphone and are meant to allow participants to connect with any of these instruments and trigger it to play some form of preferred stimulation by means of small/simple motor responses. In practice, the participant can use the microswitch as a request tool and can get the requests satisfied by the computer, smartphone, or tablet connected to the microswitch in a direct and independent manner (Roche et al., 2015; Tam et al., 2011). Two studies (Lancioni et al., 2022c, 2022a) are here summarized to clarify how microswitch-based programs can be used.

Study 1

In this study, Lancioni et al. (2022c) provided each of the 10 participants (one adolescent and nine adults) with two different microswitches. This meant that the participants could use either microswitch (expectedly the one that was more convenient for them to activate at each response occasion) to make their requests for (and then access) their preferred stimulation. Specifically, the technology involved a smartphone with Android operating system, which was (a) fitted with the MacroDroid application (i.e., an application serving to control the smartphone's functioning during the program) and (b) linked through a special interface to the two microswitches available for each participant. The microswitches, which varied across participants to suit their motor condition, included pressure and touch sensors as well as optic (proximity) sensors. Each microswitch activation (request) was followed by the smartphone's delivery of 10 s of stimulation considered to be preferred by the participants. The results showed that all participants increased their response/request frequency and thus were able to independently increase their access to preferred stimulation. Several participants used both microswitches for their requests. Other participants seemed to concentrate more on one of the microswitches. The data also showed that all participants displayed indices of satisfaction/happiness during the program.

Study 2

In the second study, Lancioni et al. (2022a) worked with 12 participants (all adults). The goal of the study was to allow the participants to request and access two different types of preferred stimulation through the use of two adjacent microswitches. The microswitches consisted of two mini voice recording devices that could be activated by a light finger–/hand-pushing response. Each voice recording device was fitted with a simple verbal request message (e.g., "Hey Google shuffle rock" or "Hey Google shuffle voice"). When the participants activated a microswitch/voice recording device, this verbalized the request message recorded in it. This message triggered the Google Assistant of a smartphone with Android operating system. The Google Assistant in turn made the smartphone deliver a brief segment (i.e., 10 s) of the stimulation requested. The results showed that all participants were able to use the microswitches to make their requests and access both types of preferred stimulation independently. Whether access to one stimulation or the other was the result of purposeful choice is not obvious from the data. To find an answer to this question, one should have probably carried out a test during which each microswitch could be intermittently connected to highly preferred or neutral (low-preference) stimuli as done in a study (Lancioni et al., 2008) reviewed below (see Sect. 3: "Programs Involving the Use of Microswitches Combined with Voice Output Devices to Enable People with Severe Post-Coma Conditions to Make Requests" focused on programs for post-coma people with extensive neuromotor and cognitive disabilities).

Section 2: Programs Involving the Use of Two Microswitches to Allow People with Severe/Profound Intellectual and Sensory-Motor Disabilities or Severe Post-Coma Conditions to Access Environmental Stimulation and Ask for Caregiver Attention

While the programs described in the previous section were directed at enabling the participants to request/access preferred environmental stimulation, the programs reported in this section were aimed at providing participants with two different opportunities, that is, (a) an opportunity to request for and access preferred stimulation directly via the technology system available, and (b) an opportunity to ask for caregiver attention and thus access forms of verbal and physical interaction with the caregiver. The three studies summarized below provide examples of how those programs can be implemented, a view of their potential impact in increasing the participants' positive activation, and a prospect of what social raters think about their effectiveness, friendliness to participants, and overall applicability in daily contexts.

Study 1

In the first of the three studies, Lancioni et al. (2009b) assessed a program with eight participants (children and adolescents) with severe/profound intellectual and sensory-motor disabilities. The technology included touch, pressure, and tilt microswitches that could be activated with simple head and arm/hand responses. Each participant was provided with one microswitch that they could use to request stimulation that was automatically delivered via an electronic control system as well as a microswitch that was combined with a voice output apparatus. Activation of the second microswitch led to the verbalization of a request to the caregiver (e.g., "Can you play with me?"). This verbalization was then followed by the caregiver responding with positive verbal and physical attention. The program involved three intervention phases, that is, one in which the participants had the microswitch for accessing preferred stimulation from the electronic system, a second in which the participants had the microswitch combined with the vocal output apparatus for requesting caregiver attention, and a third in which both types of microswitch were available. All participants learned to use both microswitches and, during the third phase of the intervention, made requests for their stimulation via the system as well as requests for caregiver attention. A survey of university psychology students and postgraduate clinical trainees provided high ratings of the program, its beneficial impact on participants' access to stimulation and communication events, and its friendliness and general applicability.

Study 2

Lancioni et al. (2009a) carried out a replication of the aforementioned study with 11 participants (children and adolescents). The new study included the same phases as the previous one plus a postintervention check to determine the stability of the participants' performance over time. The results were largely in line with those reported above. A social validation check involving university psychology students showed that they largely preferred the combination of the two types of microswitches (i.e., the third phase of the program) over any of the previous two phases.

Study 3

In this study, Lancioni et al. (2021) worked with eight participants (adults) who presented with severe post-coma conditions (i.e., extensive neuromotor impairments, lack of speech and cognitive disabilities due to acquired neurological disorders). The technology included an Eco Dot with Amazon Alexa, a smartphone, and two voice recording devices. Each voice recording device had a message recorded in it and the message was uttered as soon as the participants applied a light pressure on the device. The messages consisted of "Alexa music" and "Alexa call the caregiver (NAME)." In the first case, the system would respond to the participant's request by playing part of one of the songs pre-selected for that particular participant. In the second case, the system emitted a vocal call to the caregiver named in the request. The caregiver would respond to the call and pleasantly interact with the participant for about 1 min. All participants were able to use the system to ask for (and access) songs and caregiver attention. Typically, the frequency of requests for songs was higher than the requests for caregiver attention.

Section 3: Programs Involving the Use of Microswitches Combined with Voice Output Devices to Enable People with Severe Post-Coma Conditions to Make Requests

These programs were specifically aimed at enabling participants with extensive neuromotor impairments, lack of speech, and cognitive disabilities to make requests for interacting with socially and emotionally relevant partners. The range of neuromotor, speech, and cognitive disabilities the participants presented was due to traumatic events occurring at different points of their life. The two studies summarized below describe two of these cases and how the technology-aided programs set up for them supported them in building some form of communication with special communication partners.

Study 1

In the first study, Lancioni et al. (2008) worked with a 30-year-old man who had been involved in a road accident and had suffered extensive brain damage. He was in a wheelchair and could manage minimal hand and head movements. He could also produce some vocal emissions, orient his eyes to stimuli, and show smiles in relation to some of them (e.g., preferred music). The technology included (a) a touch sensor that was applied to the participant's right thumb to detect its minimal movements and (b) sound-detecting sensors. Thumb movements were followed by the delivery of brief segments of preferred music via an electronic control system linked to the touch sensor (i.e., as described in the studies reviewed above). The second type of microswitches consisted of sensors that served to monitor two different (i.e., short and long) vocal emissions. Activation of the sound-detecting sensors with a brief or a long vocal emission led a related vocal output instrument to call the participant's sister or the participant's mother (i.e., the sister when the vocal emission was brief and the mother when the vocal emission was long).

During an early phase of the study, the mother and sister responded by contacting the participant and providing him with preferred stimuli. During a subsequent phase of the study, there were two changes. The first consisted of the sister providing low-preference stimuli while the mother continued to provide highly preferred stimuli. The second consisted of having the mother provide low-preference stimuli and the sister highly preferred stimuli. The results showed that the participant increased the frequency of the thumb response as well as the frequency of vocal emissions/responses during the intervention phases of the study (i.e., compared to the baseline period). The overall frequencies of short and long vocal emissions/responses were very similar when his mother and sister provided highly preferred stimuli. The frequencies changed in favor of the long emissions (mother) when the sister provided low-preference stimuli. Vice versa, the frequencies changed in favor of the short emissions (sister) when the mother provided low-preference stimuli. In essence, the data indicated that the participant (a) used the vocal emissions to call the sister and the mother and (b) was purposeful in his calls (i.e., made clear choices based on the stimuli that the sister and his mother presented).

Study 2

In the second study, Lancioni et al. (2009) worked with a young man of 18 years of age who had suffered a traumatic head injury and was characterized by spastic tetraparesis, lack of trunk control, absence of speech, and reportedly severe cognitive disability. The technology included an optic and a tilt microswitch/sensor, which could be activated by small right-hand movement and lifting his right big toe, respectively. The microswitches were connected to voice output instruments. Activating the first microswitch (i.e., through a small hand movement) resulted in a verbal call for a research assistant who had a long and special relationship with the participant. Activating the second microswitch (i.e., through a movement of the right big toe) resulted in a verbal call for the mother or grandfather. The research assistant would respond by engaging the participant in some body movements and talking to him for about 20 s. His mother or grandfather would respond by telling him stories, showing pictures, and playing music or singing for about 20 s. The microswitches were introduced in succession and eventually were made available simultaneously. Data showed that the participant learned to activate both microswitches and had a high frequency of responses on both of them. No specific evidence was available as to whether he had preferences for one of the two or not.

Section 4: Programs Involving the Use of Specific Technology Systems to Enable People with Moderate Intellectual Disability and Sensory-Motor Impairments to Make Multiple Requests

The participants who are involved in these programs generally have a higher level of intellectual/cognitive functioning compared to those described in the previous sections. Concomitantly, the communication needs of these participants and the technology systems employed for them are also different from those described above. In practice, their communication needs are not related to one or few requests but tend to include a variety of requests for events and activities relevant to them in terms of immediate satisfaction and occupational engagement. The three studies summarized below assessed three types of programs for participants with important differences in their general conditions.

Study 1

In this study, Lancioni et al. (2016) worked with three adults who were considered to function in the mild-to-moderate or moderate-to-severe range of intellectual disability and also presented with sensory and motor impairments. Specifically, two of them were diagnosed with blindness and deafness plus motor impairment. The third had minimal residual vision and motor impairment. All three participants were involved in a number of occupational and recreational activities during the day (e.g., being guided to the coffee machine and drinking coffee, accessing preferred food items, sorting or assembling objects, and receiving sport news). However, they did not have effective means to request those activities. In fact, they lacked speech and their use of few gestures or object/picture cues did not attract staff or caregivers' attention when staff or caregivers were not in the immediate context (i.e., in their proximity). The study's aim was to develop and assess a special speech-generating system that could be suitable for use by these participants and other people with similar characteristics. Such system included a battery-powered computer fitted inside a box-like structure of 35 × 20 × 4 cm. The 35 × 20 cm structure's side facing the participants was divided into 15 squares of 5 × 5 cm. Each square contained a hidden optic sensor that was covered by (a) a small object representing a specific activity (e.g., a small cup representing coffee drinking at the coffee machine, and a small ball representing receiving football news) or (b) a small tag with an activity name written in Braille. The small objects and tags were fixed onto the system with Velcro. By removing an object or a tag, the participant would activate the underlying optic sensor. This operation made the sensor send a signal to the computer. The computer in turn verbalized the request matching the signal (matching the object removed). Such verbalization was audible for staff and caregivers available in the context. In response to any verbalization, staff/caregivers would approach the participant and ensure that the request being made via computer was satisfied.

The results showed that the mean frequency of requests made by the three participants during 1-hour sessions was 6, 10, and 11. The time for making the requests and carrying out the related activities was between 45 and 50 min per session. Thus, the participants remained largely busy throughout the sessions. A preference check in which the participants were made to choose between having a session with the system and engaging in a daily occupational activity showed that the participants had a preference for the sessions with the system. Finally, a staff survey about the system and its impact showed that staff had very favorable ratings.

Study 2

In this study, Lancioni et al. (2023b) assessed a program that involved the use of a new upgraded technology solution compared to the one described above. Six adults were involved in the study. Two of them were blind and deaf while the others had visual impairments that varied from functional residual vision to blindness. The technology used with them included a smartphone fitted with MacroDroid application and cardboard chips fitted with a picture (for participants who had sufficient residual vision) or a mini object (for the other participants). The cardboard chips were fitted with radio-frequency identification tags. The MacroDroid application was used to (a) ensure that the smartphone would recognize the cardboard chips (i.e., by having its Near Field Communication module discriminate the tags attached to the chips) and (b) make the smartphone verbalize the requests connected to the cardboard chips as soon as it recognized/discriminated the tags attached to them.

In practice, each participant was provided with a smartphone and nine cardboard chips at the start of every 20-min session. The smartphone was fixed on the desk at which the participant sat, at the participant's chest, or on the participant's leg. The cardboard chips were on the desk or in a bag that could be tied at the participant's belt or on the chair. To make a request, the participants were to take one of the cardboard chips and bring it into contact with the smartphone. As soon as the cardboard chip was recognized by the smartphone's Near Field Communication module, the MacroDroid application triggered the smartphone to (a) provide a vibratory feedback to the participant and (b) verbalize the request connected to that specific cardboard chip. Each request was then satisfied by providing participants with the requested stimuli. Delivery and consumption of drink and food items could be completed fairly rapidly. Some occupational activities on the contrary could last several minutes and also include the involvement of staff personnel. Data showed that all participants learned to use the system to make requests. Their mean frequency of requests per session varied between about 4.5 and 10. A staff survey on the system provided high ratings about its suitability, friendliness, effectiveness, and usability within daily contexts.

Study 3

In this final study, Lancioni et al. (2024a) worked with a man who presented with blindness, deafness, lack of speech, extensive motor impairment (i.e., he was in a wheelchair and his left arm could move only minimally), and tactile discrimination problems. These problems made it difficult for the man to recognize objects based on the manipulation of them. He was able to make a number of one-hand signs, but their use was not adequate to call staff and caregivers' attention when these were not in his proximity. Thus, signs were not considered to be an effective means for him to make requests within his daily context. The study was directed at assessing two technology systems that would enable the man's one-hand signs to produce verbal messages/requests audible to staff and caregivers regardless of whether they were in his proximity or not. One of the systems included nine mini recording devices that were fixed on the man's clothes and his wheelchair, could be reached by the man while making specific movements (e.g., touching his shoulders, his legs, or the extremities of his wheelchair's armrest), and could be activated by light hand pressure. Each of those devices contained a recorded message (request). By making specific movements and touching the devices, the man could activate those messages (i.e., could make clearly audible verbal requests).

The other system included nine tags with radio-frequency identification codes, a smartphone, and a tag reader linked via Bluetooth to the smartphone. The tags were fixed in approximately the same positions as the mini recording devices used by the first system, so they could be reached comfortably. The tag reader was worn by the man on his wrist. Each tag was programmed to represent a specific message/request. Requests were recognized by the tag reader when the man made the movement related to it (i.e., thus reaching the tag with his wrist and tag reader). Recognition of a tag's message led the tag reader to activate the smartphone and make it verbalize the message. Data showed that the man made a mean of about 10 requests per 20-min session during the intervention periods in which the first technology system was available. During the sessions in which the man used the second technology system, the mean frequency of request per session was very similar. The relatively high frequencies of requests seemed to be mainly connected to the fact that several of those requests (e.g., requests for food items or interactive games) could be satisfied in a relatively short period of time.

Section 5: Programs Involving the Use of Specific Technology Systems to Enable People with Moderate Intellectual Disability and Sensory-Motor Impairments to Engage in Video Calls and Other Activities

The two studies and related programs summarized in this section were directed at people with moderate intellectual disability and sensory-motor impairments and presented two main differences compared to those examined above. The first difference was that the form of communication targeted was not making requests as in previous studies, but rather getting in touch with distant partners (e.g., family members) preferably via video calls. The second difference was that communication was not the only focus of the programs. Specifically, the programs were also designed to include other relevant areas in which people had serious difficulties (e.g., recreational occupation or combinations of recreational occupation and functional task engagement).

Study 1

In this study, Lancioni et al. (2020) worked with eight adults who presented with moderate intellectual disability coupled with sensory and/or motor impairments as well as lack of expressive or expressive and receptive verbal skills. The goal of the study was to enable these participants to access video calls with distant partners (e.g., family and staff members not present in their immediate environment) and forms of leisure engagement. The technology consisted of a tablet with Android operating system, front camera, proximity sensor, and multimedia player. The tablet was fitted with a SIM card, the WhatsApp messenger application for making video calls, and the MacroDroid application for programming and regulating the tablet's functioning. At the start of every program session, the tablet presented three pictures representing leisure events and three pictures representing preferred partners. The pictures were scanned/lit in sequence, 5 s per picture. The participant could select a leisure event or a partner to reach via video call by touching or approaching the tablet's proximity sensor in concomitance with the picture of that event or partner being lit.

Selection of a leisure event led the tablet to present one of the preferred options being available for it (e.g., one of the participant's preferred comic videos that had been stored in the tablet). Selection of a partner led the tablet to initiate a video call with that partner via WhatsApp Messenger. The leisure events would play for about 1.5 min. The video calls did not have time restrictions. At the end of a leisure event or video call, the tablet presented a new choice opportunity following the same process described above. Sessions were scheduled to last 10 min. The results indicate that all participants were able to use the technology successfully to select leisure events and make video calls. Specifically, they spent between 30 and 55% of the session time engaging in leisure events and between 25 and 50% of the session time in video calls with preferred partners. Their cumulative occupation time covered 75–90% of the session length.

Study 2

In this second study, Lancioni et al. (2022b) worked with four adults who were diagnosed with moderate intellectual disability, motor impairment (two of them were nonambulatory), and sensory impairment (two had blindness or reduced visual acuity and two had hearing loss). The objective of the study was to enable the participants to independently (a) set up communication exchanges with distant partners through video calls (vocal calls for the participant with blindness), (b) access preferred leisure events, and (c) carry out functional tasks. The technology included a smartphone or tablet combined with a twin switch device and a mini speaker. The smartphone and tablet were provided with a SIM card, Internet connection, and WhatsApp and MacroDroid applications. At the start of a session, the system informed via the mini speaker or via images on the tablet screen that they could listen to music or watch videos by pressing one of the switches (the one with rough/green cover) and could call a preferred partner by pressing the other switch (the one with smooth/red cover). By pressing the first/leisure switch, they were presented with names of singers or images of videos. Pressing the same switch when a specific singer's name or the image of a specific video was indicated led the system to present a song of that singer or a video matching that image. Song and video were played for about 1.5 min. Pressing the second/communication switch led the system to present the names or show the images, of different communication partners. Pressing the same switch after a specific name/image led the system to start a video call (audio call for the blind participant) with the corresponding partner. At the end of a song/video or call, the system typically offered the participants a new choice opportunity by following the same process described above. Thereafter, the system was set to present the step instructions for a functional task. This could consist of collecting objects from different areas or using the objects available at the participants' desk to complete different object kits. Following the task, the system provided the participants with a new leisure/communication choice period (i.e., identical to the one described above). In practice, a session included four leisure/communication choice periods interspersed with three different tasks. Results showed that the participants used the technology successfully during sessions that lasted between 24 and 41 min. During those sessions, the participants accessed a mean of about 4.5–6 leisure events and a mean of 2.3–3.3 calls. Moreover, the mean percentage of task steps correctly performed was about or above 98.

Section 6: Conditions Necessary to Make the Programs and Technology Solutions Reviewed Above Applicable and Effective

The programs and related technologies described in this chapter are means to help people with intellectual and motor or sensory-motor disabilities and may be applicable and effective provided that at least two critical conditions are met. The first necessary condition is the existence of a reasonable match between the participants' intellectual and sensory-motor functioning and the scope of the program. The second condition to be met is a correspondence (an adequate match) between the participants' motor and visual skills and the responses required by the technology adopted in the program.

As it may be clear from the studies reviewed, the participants' level of intellectual functioning and their motor or sensory-motor condition are the main variables that determine the type of program and technology that one may use with them. For a number of participants who present with severe/profound intellectual/cognitive disability and extensive motor impairment (with or without sensory impairments), the option available is a program relying on the use of one or two microswitches linked to one or two responses that the participants are apparently able to control (Lancioni et al., 2012, 2022c; Roche et al., 2015; Shih & Shih, 2010). For these participants, the use of the microswitch(es) may be a viable way to make basic stimulation requests and have such requests automatically satisfied by the technology system being employed, that is, the computer, tablet, or smartphone interfaced to the microswitch(es).

For other participants with a diagnosis of severe/profound intellectual (cognitive) disability and sensory-motor impairments, more program options may be available. Those options may involve the use of (a) two microswitches, each allowing the participants to request for a specific type of preferred stimulation and automatically access each of the two stimulation alternatives through the technology system available, (b) one microswitch allowing the request and automatic access to preferred stimulation and one microswitch combined with a voice output device allowing the request for caregiver attention, and (c) two microswitches combined with voice output devices to make requests for the attention interaction with different relevant partners (e.g., family members or staff persons) (Lancioni et al., 2008, 2009b, b, 2022a). With some of these participants, one might even alternate sessions in which microswitches allow automatic access to stimulation with sessions in which the microswitches are combined with voice output devices allowing requests for contact with different staff and caregivers available in the context. The first type of sessions could be arranged in situations in which staff and caregivers are not able to ensure interaction with the participants. The second type of sessions could be arranged in situations in which staff and caregivers are able to respond to the participants' requests.

Participants with moderate intellectual disability and motor or sensory-motor impairments would generally be able to make a larger number of requests compared to the participants mentioned above and thus the intervention programs would need to focus on providing them the opportunity to make those requests in a feasible and effective manner. For some of these participants, one may (a) conceive the use of programs directed at enabling them to make visual and auditory contact with relevant people who are not present in the context (Lancioni et al., 2022c), and (b) eventually extend those programs to include other important aspects of the participants' life such as leisure engagement and performance of functional daily tasks (Lancioni et al., 2022c, b, 2023a).

The success of an intervention program would generally depend on whether its purpose is fitting the participants' functioning level and on whether the technology adopted suits the participants' sensory-motor conditions. For example, participants with extensive motor impairment may not necessarily possess responses such as hand-pushing, which can be easily detected via various types of pressure microswitches/sensors (e.g., traditional pressure devices and mini recording devices). Rather, they may possess (a) motor responses such as partial hand closures that one may monitor via touch-sensitive microswitches fixed inside the participants' hand (i.e., in the palm of their hand), or (b) responses such as forehead skin movements, limited finger or toe movements, and prolonged eye closures. Monitoring these types of responses often requires the use of new forms of microswitches/sensors (e.g., optic or camera-based sensors) and/or special ways of positioning those microswitches/sensors (Lancioni et al., 2013; Mena et al., 2019; Perilli et al., 2019).

It is also the case that many people with visual or visual and motor disabilities would not be able to make multiple requests using common speech-generating devices due to the fact that the use of these devices typically requires visual discrimination and fine motor skills. Helping these people make requests can be possible only if the technology available does not require them to make fine motor responses and to rely on visual discrimination. The two studies involving people with severe cognitive disability and extensive neuromotor impairment following acquired brain injury (Lancioni et al., 2008, 2009; see Sect. 3: "Programs Involving the Use of Microswitches Combined with Voice Output Devices to Enable People with Severe Post-Coma Conditions to Make Requests") and the three studies involving people with moderate intellectual disability and sensory-motor impairments (Lancioni et al., 2016, 2023b, 2024a; see Sect. 4: "Programs Involving the Use of Specific Technology Systems to Enable People with Moderate Intellectual Disability and Sensory-Motor Impairments to Make Multiple Requests") provide some general guidelines for setting up successful programs in this area. People of the first group may require the use of specific microswitches (i.e., capable of detecting their responses even if these are small) connected to voice output devices to make basic requests for stimulation and human contact. People of the second group may need to be provided with new technology systems (i.e., alternatives to typical speech-generating devices) that are not ready-made for use but need to be set up by employing commercially available components (e.g., smartphones, mini recording devices, radio-frequency identification tags, and applications such as the MacroDroid). New technology solutions may also be employed to set up programs directed at helping people communicate with distant partners and possibly engage in leisure activities and occupational tasks.

Section 7: Accessibility and Practicality of the Programs

The accessibility and practicality of a program can be determined based on (a) the cost of the technology needed for the program, (b) the amount of work and expertise required to set up the technology for use in the program, and (c) the time that staff need to invest to set up the sessions with the program (Abdi et al., 2021; Boot et al., 2018, Borg, 2019; Botelho, 2021). With regard to the first point, the answer may be relatively encouraging. For example, the technology components required to set up a program with one or two microswitches (e.g., the microswitch or microswitches, a smartphone with an application such as the MacroDrooid, and an interface) may cost about $500. The cost may increase only slightly when the activation of the microswitches is set to produce verbal requests. In fact, the requests could be recorded in the smartphone and emitted through a mini speaker connected to the smartphone via Bluetooth. The technology components required to set up a program for multiple requests may change based on the type of program chosen. The simplest of the three programs summarized in this chapter (see Lancioni et al., 2023b) includes a smartphone, cardboard chips fitted with radio-frequency identification tags, a special application such as the MacroDroid, and a mini speaker. The cost for such a package may be about $400. The components for a program allowing the participants to access video calls with distant partners and leisure events, and to carry out functional multistep activities would include a tablet with a SIM card and WhatsApp and MacroDroid applications, specific response switches, and an interface. The cost of this particular package could be about or slightly more than $600.

None of the technology packages mentioned above or reviewed earlier in the chapter is a commercial product ready for use within a program. While the technology components can easily be purchased, their functioning within the program depends on the setting up of the smartphone or tablet being used and the programming of those devices through the special application available (e.g., MacroDroid). Such programming is aimed at determining what the smartphone/tablet would present to the participants and how it would respond to the participants' input through the means they have available (e.g., response switches and cardboard chips fitted with radio-frequency identification tags). Such programming, albeit not too complex, may not be manageable by staff or caregivers have less familiarity with such technology. This may limit the accessibility and usability of the programs in situations in which these staff and caregivers do not have adequate technological support.

Once the technology required for a program has been adequately prepared, setting up program sessions may be relatively simple and practically viable. The staff time investment during the sessions would depend on the nature of the program. Programs enabling the participants to make requests for caregiver attention or specific items/activities demand that staff and caregivers are available to respond to those requests (Lancioni et al., 2016, 2023b). Programs focused on supporting the participants to access leisure events, perform functional activities, and communicate (interact) with distant partners would require no specific staff presence during the sessions (Lancioni et al., 2022b).

Section 8: Perspectives on the Use of the Programs over Time

Technology-aided programs may sometimes be considered temporary aids (i.e., as aids to help the participants acquire skills that would then make them independent) (Lancioni et al., 2024d). Yet, technology-aided programs set up to help participants with intellectual and sensory-motor disabilities access communication events such as those described in this chapter may be viewed as long-term aids (i.e., as prosthetic tools) (Halvorsrud et al. 2023; Horton 2021; Mishra et al., 2022). The participants would not be expected to develop skills that could make them reach their communication aims without the support of the technology available in those programs. For example, one cannot envisage people with extensive motor impairment and lack of speech to acquire the ability to make requests independent of some of the support means described in the chapter. Their conditions in fact would not be expected to have sufficiently large types of improvement over time (Howard et al. 2022; Hoyle et al. 2020; Nakayama 2023, Smith et al., 2021).

Realizing that the technology-aided programs may be a long-term means can be taken as a prompt and incentive to upgrade the resources presently available and develop new ones with the aim of making them more easily accessible and programmable. Improving accessibility and reducing programming requirements can help extend the acceptance and usability of technology-aided programs across a wider range of education and rehabilitation contexts.

Summary and Conclusion

The chapter has reviewed a number of technology-aided programs carried out with people with intellectual disability (or cognitive disability following traumatic brain injury) combined with extensive motor or sensory-motor impairments. The programs' outcomes may be considered encouraging as to the possibility of helping a group of people for whom conventional intervention programs and technology solutions may have limited applicability. It was also underlined that the effectiveness of the programs may require two basic conditions: (a) a reasonable match between the participants' intellectual and sensory-motor functioning and the scope of the program, and (b) a correspondence (an adequate match) between the participants' motor and visual skills and the response requirements of the technology adopted in the program. The accessibility of the technology used in the programs seems to be relatively high in terms of costs. Yet, the technology is not ready-made for use and thus some technical skills are required from staff to set it up. This skill requirement may be a point to consider in preparing staff personnel to work in this area. One last point that needs attention because of its large practical implications is that the use of these programs may hardly be considered a temporary commitment. The general motor and sensory conditions of the participants to whom those programs are directed cannot be really expected to improve and allow the participants to become independent of the programs over time.

References

Abdi, S., Kitsara, I., Hawley, M. S., & de Witte, L. P. (2021). Emerging technologies and their potential for generating new assistive technologies. *Assistive Technology, 33*(sup1), 17–26. https://doi.org/10.1080/10400435.2021.1945704

Badia, M., Orgaz, M. B., Verdugo, M. A., & Ullán, A. M. (2013). Patterns and determinants of leisure participation of youth and adults with developmental disabilities. *Journal of Intellectual Disability Research, 57*(4), 319–332. https://doi.org/10.1111/j.1365-2788.2012.01539.x

Boot, F. H., Owuor, J., Dinsmore, J., & MacLachlan, M. (2018). Access to assistive technology for people with intellectual disabilities: A systematic review to identify barriers and facilitators. *Journal of Intellectual Disability Research, 62*(10), 900–921. https://doi.org/10.1111/jir.12532

Borg, J. (2019). Commentary on selection of assistive technology in a context with limited resources. *Disability and Rehabilitation: Assistive Technology, 14*(8), 753–754. https://doi.org/10.1080/17483107.2019.1657188

Botelho, F. H. F. (2021). Accessibility to digital technology: Virtual barriers, real opportunities. *Assistive Technology, 33*(sup1), 27–34. https://doi.org/10.1080/10400435.2021.1945705

Burns, J., Carter, A., Draper, S., & Foad, A. (2022). Engaging and sustaining people with intellectual disabilities in physical activity: A narrative review of existing evidence. *International Journal of Developmental Disabilities, 70*(5), 803–813. https://doi.org/10.1080/20473869.2022.2149096

Chan, J. M., Lambdin, L., Van Laarhoven, T., & Johnson, J. W. (2013). Teaching leisure skills to an adult with developmental disabilities using a video prompting intervention package. *Education and Training in Autism and Developmental Disabilities, 48*(3), 412–420. http://www.jstor.org/stable/23880997

Danker, J., Dreyfus, S., Strnadovà, I., & Pilkinton, M. (2023). Scoping review on communication systems used by adults withsevere/profound intellectual disability for functional communication. *Journal of Applied Research in Intellectual Disabilities, 36*(5), 951–965. https://doi.org/10.1111/jar.13133

Darcy, S., Green, J., & Maxwell, H. (2017). I've got a mobile phone too! Hard and soft assistive technology customization and supportive call centres for people with disability. *Disability and Rehabilitation: Assistive Technology, 12*(4), 341–351. https://doi.org/10.3109/17483107.2016.1167260

Desideri, L., Lancioni, G., Malavasi, M., Gherardini, A., & Cesario, L. (2021). Step-instruction technology to help people with intellectual and other disabilities perform multistep tasks: A literature review. *Journal of Developmental and Physical Disabilities, 33*(3), 857–886. https://doi.org/10.1007/s10882-020-09781-7

Dijkhuizen, A., Hilgenkamp, T. I., Krijnen, W. P., van der Schans, C. P., & Waninge, A. (2016). The impact of visual impairment on the ability to perform activities of daily living for persons with severe/profound intellectual disability. *Research in Developmental Disabilities, 48*, 35–42. https://doi.org/10.1016/j.ridd.2015.10.001

Halvorsrud, L., Holthe, T., Karterud, D., Thorstensen, E., & Lund, A. (2023). Perspectives on assistive technology among older Norwegian adults receiving community health services. *Disability and Rehabilitation: Assistive Technology, 18*(5), 685–692. https://doi.org/10.1080/17483107.2021.1906962

Hassan, N. M., Landorf, K. B., Shields, N., & Munteanu, S. E. (2019). Effectiveness of interventions to increase physical activity in individuals with intellectual disabilities: A systematic review of randomised controlled trials. *Journal of Intellectual Disability Research, 63*(2), 168–191. https://doi.org/10.1111/jir.12562

Horton, S. (2021). Empathy cannot sustain action in technology accessibility. *Frontiers in Computer Science, 3*, 617044. https://doi.org/10.3389/fcomp.2021.617044

Howard, J., Fisher, Z., Kemp, A. H., Lindsay, S., Tasker, L. H., & Tree, J. J. (2022). Exploring the barriers to using assistive technology for individuals with chronic conditions: A meta-synthesis

review. *Disability and Rehabilitation. Assistive Technology, 17*(4), 390–408. https://doi.org/10.1080/17483107.2020.1788181
Hoyle, J. N., Laditka, J. N., & Laditka, S. B. (2020). Severe developmental disability and the transition to adulthood. *Disability and Health Journal, 13*(3), 100912. https://doi.org/10.1016/j.dhjo.2020.100912
Kotloski, R. J., & Sutula, T. P. (2015). Environmental enrichment: Evidence for an unexpected therapeutic influence. *Experimental Neurology, 264*, 121–126. https://doi.org/10.1016/j.expneurol.2014.11.012
Lancioni, G. E., Alberti, G., Filippini, C., Singh, N. N., O'Reilly, M., & Sigafoos, J. (2024c). A technology-aided program to help people with profound intellectual and multiple disabilities access preferred stimulation and exercise motor responses and visual orientation. *OBM Neurobiology, 8*(2), 228. https://doi.org/10.21926/obm.neurobiol.2402228
Lancioni, G. E., Alberti, G., Pezzuoli, F., Bruciati, J., Singh, N. N., O'Reilly, M., & Sigafoos, J. (2024a). Technology systems to enable a man with intellectual, sensory and motor disabilities to make verbal requests through simple one-hand signs: Proof-of-concept study. *Journal of Enabling Technologies, 18*(1), 50–58. https://doi.org/10.1108/JET-08-2023-0028
Lancioni, G. E., Bellini, D., Oliva, D., Singh, N. N., O'Reilly, M. F., Sigafoos, J., & Lang, R. (2012). Two persons with multiple disabilities use camera-based microswitch technology to control stimulation with small mouth and eyelid responses. *Journal of Intellectual and Developmental Disabilities, 37*(4), 337–342. https://doi.org/10.3109/13668250.2012.726351
Lancioni, G. E., O'Reilly, M. F., Sigafoos, J., D'Amico, F., Spica, A., Buonocunto, F., Del Gaudio, V., Lanzilotti, C., & Navarro, J. (2021). Mainstream technology as basic support for individuals with extensive neuro-motor impairments and absence of verbal skills. *Advances in Neurodevelopmental Disorders, 5*(1), 85–92. https://doi.org/10.1007/s41252-020-00183-6
Lancioni, G. E., O'Reilly, M. F., Singh, N. N., Buonocunto, F., Sacco, V., Colonna, F., Navarro, J., Oliva, D., Megna, G., & Bosco, A. (2009). Technology-based intervention options for post-coma persons with minimally conscious state and pervasive motor disabilities. *Developmental Neurorehabilitation, 12*(1), 24–31. https://doi.org/10.1080/17518420902776995
Lancioni, G. E., O'Reilly, M. F., Singh, N. N., Sigafoos, J., Didden, R., Oliva, D., Campodonico, F., De Pace, C., Chiapparino, C., & Groeneweg, J. (2009a). Persons with multiple disabilities accessing stimulation and requesting social contact via microswitch and VOCA devices: New research evaluation and social validation. *Research in Developmental Disabilities, 30*(5), 1084–1094. https://doi.org/10.1016/j.ridd.2009.03.004
Lancioni, G. E., O'Reilly, M. F., Singh, N. N., Sigafoos, J., Oliva, D., Smaldone, A., La Martire, M. L., Antonucci, M., De Pace, C., & Chiapparino, C. (2009b). Persons with multiple disabilities access stimulation and contact the caregiver via microswitch and VOCA technology. *Life Span and Disability, 22*(2), 119–128.
Lancioni, G. E., Olivetti Belardinelli, M., Stasolla, F., Singh, N. N., O'Reilly, M., Sigafoos, J., & Angelillo, M. T. (2008). Promoting engagement, requests and choice by a man with post-coma pervasive motor impairment and minimally conscious state through a technology-based program. *Journal of Developmental and Physical Disabilities, 20*(4), 379–388. https://doi.org/10.1007/s10882-008-9104-x
Lancioni, G. E., Sigafoos, J., O'Reilly, M. F., & Singh, N. N. (2013). *Assistive technology: Interventions for individuals with severe/profound and multiple disabilities*. Springer.
Lancioni, G. E., Singh, N. N., O'Reilly, M. F., Green, V. A., van der Meer, L., Alberti, G., Perilli, V., Boccasini, A., La Martire, M. L., & Lang, R. (2016). A speech generating device for persons with intellectual and sensory-motor disabilities. *Journal of Developmental and Physical Disabilities, 28*(1), 85–98. https://doi.org/10.1007/s10882-015-9424-6
Lancioni, G. E., Singh, N. N., O'Reilly, M. F., & Sigafoos, J. (2024d). Possible assistive technology solutions for people with moderate to severe/profound intellectual and multiple disabilities: Considerations on their function and long-term role. *International Journal of Developmental Disabilities*. https://doi.org/10.1080/20473869.2024.2303532

Lancioni, G. E., Singh, N. N., O'Reilly, M. F., Sigafoos, J., Alberti, G., Campodonico, F., Acquaviva, G., Chiariello, V., & Desideri, L. (2022a). Persons with intellectual and multiple disabilities activate via non-verbal responses a smartphone's Google assistant to access preferred stimulation. *International Journal of Developmental Disabilities, 68*(4), 518–527. https://doi.org/10.1080/20473869.2020.1827213

Lancioni, G. E., Singh, N. N., O'Reilly, M. F., Sigafoos, J., Alberti, G., Campodonico, F., & Desideri, L. (2023a). A smartphone-based program enabling people with intellectual and other disabilities to access leisure, communication, and functional activities. *Universal Access in the Information Society, 22*(4), 581–590. https://doi.org/10.1007/s10209-021-00858-4

Lancioni, G. E., Singh, N. N., O'Reilly, M. F., Sigafoos, J., Alberti, G., & Fiore, A. (2022b). People with intellectual and multiple disabilities access leisure, communication, and daily activities *via* a new technology-aided program. *Frontiers in Psychology, 13*, 994416. https://doi.org/10.3389/fpsyg.2022.994416

Lancioni, G. E., Singh, N. N., O'Reilly, M. F., Sigafoos, J., Alberti, G., Chiariello, V., & Desideri, L. (2022c). A microswitch-aided program to enable people with extensive multiple disabilities to control environmental stimulation through different responses. *Frontiers in Psychiatry, 13*, 1073650. https://doi.org/10.3389/fpsyt.2022.1073650

Lancioni, G. E., Singh, N. N., O'Reilly, M. F., Sigafoos, J., Alberti, G., Perilli, V., Chiariello, V., Grillo, G., & Turi, C. (2020). A tablet-based program to enable people with intellectual and other disabilities to access leisure activities and video calls. *Disability and Rehabilitation: Assistive Technology, 15*(1), 14–20. https://doi.org/10.1080/17483107.2018.1508515

Lancioni, G. E., Singh, N. N., O'Reilly, M. F., Sigafoos, J., Alberti, G., Troccoli, O., Orlando, I., & Ricci, C. (2023b). Enabling people with intellectual and other disabilities to make verbal requests using cardboard chips with mini objects or pictures and a smartphone. *Frontiers in Rehabilitation Sciences, 4*, 1257493. https://doi.org/10.3389/fresc.2023.1257493

Maes, B., Nijs, S., Vandesande, S., Van Keer, I., Arthur-Kelly, M., Dind, J., Goldbart, J., Petitpierre, G., & Van der Putten, A. (2021). Looking back, looking forward: Methodological challenges and future directions in research on persons with profound intellectual and multiple disabilities. *Journal of Applied Research in Intellectual Disabilities, 34*(1), 250–262. https://doi.org/10.1111/jar.12803

Mena, L. J., Felix, V. G., Ostos, R., & Maestre, G. E. (2019). Emerging technology for students with intellectual disability. In J. L. Matson (Ed.), *Handbook of intellectual disabilities: Integrating theory, research, and practice* (pp. 795–810). Springer. https://doi.org/10.1007/978-3-030-20843-1_43

Mishra, S., Laplante-Levesque, A., Barbareschi, G., De Witte, L., Abdi, S., Spann, A., Khasnabis, C., & Allen, M. (2022). Assistive technology needs, access and coverage, and related barriers and facilitators in the WHO European region: A scoping review. *Disability and Rehabilitation: Assistive Technology, 19*(2), 474–485. https://doi.org/10.1080/17483107.2022.2099021

Munde, V., & Vlaskamp, C. (2015). Initiation of activities and alertness in individuals with profound intellectual and multiple disabilities. *Journal of Intellectual Disability Research, 59*(3), 284–292. https://doi.org/10.1111/jir.12138

Nakayama, Y. (2023). Conceptual framework for understanding the transition of children with severe motor and intellectual disabilities to adult life after graduation. *International Journal of Disability, Development and Education, 70*(2), 213–227. https://doi.org/10.1080/1034912X.2020.1843605

Nijs, S., & Maes, B. (2021). Assistive technology for persons with profound intellectual disability: A European survey on attitudes and beliefs. *Disability and Rehabilitation. Assistive Technology, 16*(5), 497–504. https://doi.org/10.1080/17483107.2019.1668973

Perilli, V., Stasolla, F., & Boccasini, A. (2019). Technological solutions for helping adaptive responding of children with severe to profound developmental disabilities: A literature overview. *International Journal of Computers in Clinical Practice (IJCCP), 4*(1), 9–21. https://doi.org/10.4018/IJCCP.2019010102

Ricci, C., Miglino, O., Alberti, G., Perilli, V., & Lancioni, G. E. (2017). Speech generating technology to support request responses of persons with intellectual and multiple disabilities. *International Journal of Developmental Disabilities, 63*(4), 238–245. https://doi.org/10.1080/20473869.2017.1288888

Roche, L., Sigafoos, J., Lancioni, G. E., O'Reilly, M. F., & Green, V. A. (2015). Microswitch technology for enabling self-determined responding in children with profound and multiple disabilities: A systematic review. *Augmentative and Alternative Communication, 31*(3), 246–258. https://doi.org/10.3109/07434618.2015.1024888

Rushton, R., Kossyvaki, L., & Terlektsi, E. (2023). Music-based interventions for people with profound and multiple learning disabilities: A systematic review of the literature. *Journal of Intellectual Disabilities, 27*(2), 370–387. https://doi.org/10.1177/17446295221087563

Shih, C. H., & Shih, C. T. (2010). Assisting two children with multiple disabilities and minimal motor skills control environmental stimuli with thumb poke through a trackball. *Behavioural and Cognitive Psychotherapy, 38*(2), 211–219. https://doi.org/10.1017/S1352465809990683

Smith, E., Sumner, P., Hedge, C., & Powell, G. (2021). Smart speaker devices can improve speech intelligibility in adults with intellectual disability. *International Journal of Language & Communication Disorders, 56*(3), 583–593. https://doi.org/10.1111/1460-6984.12615

Tam, G. M., Phillips, K. J., & Mudford, O. C. (2011). Teaching individuals with profound multiple disabilities to access preferred stimuli with multiple microswitches. *Research in Developmental Disabilities, 32*(6), 2352–2361. https://doi.org/10.1016/j.ridd.2011.07.027

Ten Brug, A., Van der Putten, A. A., Penne, A., Maes, B., & Vlaskamp, C. (2016). Making a difference? A comparison between multi-sensory and regular storytelling for persons with profound intellectual and multiple disabilities. *Journal of Intellectual Disability Research, 60*(11), 1043–1053. https://doi.org/10.1111/jir.12260

Chapter 10
Visual Strategies for Receptive Communication

Introduction

This chapter focuses on the use of visual supports to enhance the receptive communication skills of individuals with severe disabilities who have limited or no speech. Receptive communication essentially involves a person's ability to understand vocabulary, syntax, and pragmatics. Individuals with extensive support needs can exhibit severe delays with learning to use words to identify items and activities (vocabulary), combining these words into meaningful sentences (syntax), and navigating the social/communicative nuances of interactions (pragmatics). As considered in earlier chapters of this book, a predominant focus of communication intervention with this population has been to teach expressive communication skills. For example, the primary focus of the research-based interventions described in Chaps. 6 and 7 was to teach individuals with severe disabilities to indicate by touching, pointing to, or exchanging objects or pictures to request items and activities.

Much of the clinical application and research to enhance receptive communication skills involves the use of aided forms of augmentative and alternative communication (AAC). Research on teaching receptive communication skills to individuals with severe disabilities and little or no speech has, in some respects, lagged behind the research on teaching expressive skills. Additionally, research addressing interventions to teach receptive communication skills is somewhat scattered with separate bodies of work focusing on vocabulary comprehension while other researchers have focused on the pragmatics of navigating social contexts (e.g., Allen et al., 2017; Arthur-Kelly et al., 2009).

J. Sigafoos et al., *Communication Strategies for People with Severe Disabilities*, Autism and Child Psychopathology Series,
https://doi.org/10.1007/978-3-031-83807-1_10

Overview of Receptive Communication Strategies and Intervention Research

Three important interventions to enhance receptive communication skills include (a) augmented input, (b) Social Stories™, and (c) the use of visual activity schedules. All three of these receptive communication strategies involve aided AAC. Augmented input focuses on teaching the learner to comprehend vocabulary, whereas Social Stories™ and visual activity schedules tend to focus on supporting social and broader contextual understanding. Each of these three intervention strategies, including illustrations from intervention research, will be described. The research studies included in this descriptive overview are summarized in Table 10.1 according to each study's setting, participants, intervention procedures, and outcomes.

Table 10.1 Summary of six intervention studies evaluating visual strategies for receptive communication

Study	Setting	Participants	Intervention	Outcome
Chan and O'Reilly (2008)	Inclusive classroom	2 autistic boys (aged 5 and 6 years)	Social stories™ read aloud plus roleplay and feedback with therapist	Increase appropriate plus decrease inappropriate social initiations with peers
Douglas et al. (2023)	Home settings	1 autistic child (aged 7 years) and 5 family members	Mother taught to train family members to use ALM* plus SGD** with child	All family members accurately implemented ALM with SGD and were positive about intervention
Drager et al. (2006)	Inclusive preschool or daycare	2 autistic children (aged 4 years)	ALM during 3 play activities with pictures of 4 targeted words per activity	Increases in receptive comprehension of pictures and objects for both children
Krantz et al. (1993)	Home settings	3 autistic children (aged 6–8 years)	Parents taught to implement individualized VAS^ in the home	Decreases in tantrums and increases in on-task behavior and social initiations
Kuttler et al. (1998)	Self-contained classroom	1 child with autism and fragile X syndrome	Social stories™ implemented prior to lunch and work periods	Reductions in tantrums during lunch and work periods at school
Morrison et al. (2002)	Inclusive preschool classroom	4 autistic children (aged 42–70 months)	VAS of 4 play activities and teacher prompted child to follow schedule	Increases in on-task behavior and schedule adherence. Decreases in problem behavior

Note. *ALM = aided language modeling. **SGD = speech-generating device. ^VAS = visual activity schedule

Augmented Input

As mentioned before, the preponderance of research on the use of aided communication strategies has focused on increasing expressive communication skills, such as requesting preferred items and activities (Crowe et al., 2022). The term augmented input is used to describe a series of instructional strategies designed to enhance both expressive and receptive communication. It has been proposed that embedding augmented input strategies as part of aided instruction can enhance learning of language form and content (Romski & Sevcik, 1997). A small body of research has focused on augmented input for learners with severe communication difficulties and comorbid diagnoses, such as intellectual disability and autism spectrum disorder (Chazin et al., 2021). Augmented input essentially involves the communication partner (e.g., teacher or parent) using natural speech coupled with input from the learner's aided communication system (e.g., pointing to relevant icons) during communication exchanges.

The impetus for using augmented input as part of aided communication intervention derives in part from observations of typical language development. In typical communication development, a child vocalizes and the parent responds through vocalization. In other words, the child receives input—such as repetition of words and phrases, acknowledgment, expansions, and recasting—through the same (auditory) communication modality. However, for learners who use aided communication strategies systems, the primary mode of expression is visual (e.g., exchanging line drawing or photographs, tapping an icon on an SGD, or touching a tangible object). In contrast, their communication input from communication partners is predominantly auditory, that is, spoken words. This creates what has been termed an input–output asymmetry, which may impede cognitive development and produce communication breakdowns between the user and his or her communication partners (Dada et al., 2021). Augmented input attempts to overcome this input–output asymmetry by pairing the selection of communication symbols used with the aided communication strategy with spoken words. The aim being to associate the spoken language with the selection of the aided communication symbols.

A variety of terminologies have been used in the research literature to describe augmented input intervention techniques (Allen et al., 2017). The common theme of these intervention techniques is that the communication partner uses speech coupled with aided input during exchanges. Examples of these augmentative intervention techniques include aided language stimulation (ALS), aided language modeling (ALM), and aided AAC modeling (AACM) (Binger & Light, 2007; Drager et al., 2006; Harris & Reichle, 2004). ALS focuses on the communication partner's use of simple phraseology with fewer words used than during typical interactions. The communication partner also expands on the learner's aided communication responses. Simultaneously, the communication partner points to the relevant symbols on the aided AAC device. ALM involves the communication partner naming an object while pointing to the corresponding picture (or other graphic representation of the item) on the aided device. The partner also points to the targeted item in the environment and then immediately points to the picture of the item on the aided device. AACM involves labeling multiple symbols while simultaneously pointing to these symbols on the device. Complete sentences are modeled and would also be produced via activation of the SGD (see Chap. 8), if such a device were being used by the learner. Overall, there appears to be considerable overlap between each of these augmented input techniques. Additionally, augmented input interventions are generally coupled with the implementation of additional instructional strategies (e.g., time delay, response prompting, prompt fading, and reinforcement for correct responding).

Drager et al. (2006) described the ALM model of augmented input and conducted a preliminary investigation of ALM with two preschool children who attended an inclusive day care program and received special education support as part of this program. Both children were 4 years old, diagnosed with autism, had fewer than 30 functional words, and could match pictures to objects (by pointing and touching). The ALM intervention was conducted in the context of three preferred play activities (e.g., doll house, cars, and playground). Four target words, representing common labels used routinely for each activity were selected. The students did not have these words in their repertoire. For example, with the car play activity, words selected included "car," "truck," "bus," and "road." Each of the target words was represented by a colored line drawing of about 7 × 7 cm in size.

The intervention was conducted in the children's classroom either on a tabletop or on the floor. During a play activity, the play materials were freely available for the child to organize and interact with while a researcher or a member of the classroom staff followed the child's lead in play. Additionally, a communication board (about 20 × 20 cm) with pictures of the four selected words for that specific activity was placed in front of the child. The four words for each activity were randomly arranged on the board for each play session. Play sessions lasted approximately 20 min and were conducted approximately twice weekly over 5 months. During the play activity, the therapist pointed to the target object and then pointed to the line drawing while saying the spoken word. This was done four times for each targeted word during the play activity.

To measure changes in comprehension of the target words prior to the ALM intervention and then during the ALM intervention, a series of comprehension probes were conducted. These comprehension probes were conducted immediately prior to the play activity sessions. Several types of comprehension probes were used. *For comprehension of graphic and verbal stimuli* probes, an array of six toys from the play activity were presented in a row in front of the child. The experimenter then presented the line drawing plus the verbal label while saying, *Show me the* …. The line drawing was centered and placed over the array of toys. A correct response required the child to grasp or point to the correct toy. Toys and symbols were randomly arranged across comprehension probes. Probes for comprehension of verbal stimuli only and comprehension of graphic stimuli only were conducted in a similar manner as the combined graphic and verbal stimuli probes. Finally, for symbol production probes, the graphic stimuli were arranged in front of the child who was then instructed to select the correct graphic symbol for the toy presented.

The effects of the ALM intervention on comprehension were assessed using a multiple baseline design. The ALM intervention was staggered across each of the three play activities for each child. The intervention demonstrated increases in all measures of comprehension across all play activities for both children. The results suggest that ALM was effective. It also appeared to be relatively easy for parents and staff to implement and use across settings.

The ability of ALM strategies to enhance communication with families in home settings has also been examined. For example, Douglas et al. (2023) examined the use of a family-centered capacity-building intervention approach to enhance a child's use of an SGD in communication with multiple family members. Examining the uptake and use of evidence-based practices to support the use of aided communication strategies in naturalistic settings is a critical aspect of communication intervention for persons with severe disabilities. The child involved in this study was a severely autistic 7-year-old girl. She communicated primarily through sign language (approximately 20 signs) and gestures at home and also used an SGD (an iPad® with the Proloquo2Go® application), although the SGD was reportedly used infrequently. The SGD displayed about 36 high-frequency core symbols such as *HELP*. Additionally, there were approximately 200 symbols across multiple screens. The child was capable of navigating across screens on the SGD, but rarely used it in the home. The family were unfamiliar with the SGD and indicated an interest in learning how to use the SGD with the child to facilitate communication.

Five family members (i.e., the mother, brother, father, aunt, and great aunt) were coached on how to implement ALM procedures with the child. The mother was trained by a researcher to implement the ALM procedures and then she trained the other family members. Each family member selected a high-frequency activity with associated SGD words to learn how to use ALM with the child. For example, the mother chose storybook reading that took place in the living room with preferred children's books. Targeted SGD words for the mother included "*want*," "*listen*," "*look*," and "*see*." The brother, in contrast, selected playing with musical toys that occurred in the playroom and target SGD words included "*want*," "*play*," "*violin*," "*singer*," and "*headphones*." And to further illustrate, the great aunt selected snack time in the kitchen and the SGD words included "*water*," "*snack*," "*banana*," "*applesauce*," and "*crackers*."

The intervention consisted of training the family to implement the ALM procedure for the targeted activity. The ALM intervention consisted of several strategies described as *prepare, show, wait,* and *respond*. *Prepare* involved the family member problem-solving the flow of an upcoming activity and key communications to be targeted. *Show* involved placing the SGD in sight and reach of the child, communicating at the child's level of using the SGD, and using spoken language simultaneously. *Wait* focused on pausing for about 3–5 s following a family member's communication to allow the child time to respond. *Respond* emphasized responding to the child's communications by acknowledging, expanding, and fulfilling any requests. Training in ALM procedures consisted of video example, modeling, role-play, and feedback. The mother was trained to implement ALM by a researcher, and she subsequently trained the other family members to implement the procedures.

Following the family training, coaching sessions were implemented several times weekly for all family members. The mother led the coaching sessions for family members. Each coaching session included pre-observation reflection and planning, direct observation of an ALM session, post-observation feedback.

The effectiveness of the training and coaching procedure was evaluated using a multiple probe design across each family member/child dyad (e.g., mother/child, brother/child, and aunt/child). The primary measure was fidelity of implementation of the ALM procedure by each family member. Results demonstrated that each family member increased in their accurate use of the ALM procedure with the child and that the results were maintained over time. While not a primary measure, it was also reported that the child increased in her word usage during the study. All family members reported being pleased with the training procedures and claimed increased use of the SGD during regular family routines. The aunt, who did not live with the family, noted that the SGD overcame communication barriers for her as she did not understand sign language (sign language was the predominant mode of communication for the child prior to ALM training with the SGD).

Social Stories™

Social Stories™ are a popular set of strategies used in clinical and educational contexts to enhance children's functioning. Social Stories™ offer insight into the "rules of engagement" of particular social contexts that may be difficult or problematic for a person. In other words, Social Stories™ are designed to enhance understanding of a social context. Additionally, appropriate communication exemplars are provided as part of the social story to enhance successful communication, and the person can generate possible positive outcomes based on successful performance.

Social Stories™ was originally proposed as a social problem-solving strategy for autistic children (Gray, 2010; Gray & Garand, 1993). Autistic children routinely experience difficulties navigating social situations, which can lead to communication breakdown, withdrawal, and problem behavior. These difficulties may be particularly evident in inclusive contexts, such as a regular classroom or playground settings where social dynamics and classroom routines can be fluid. Autistic children have difficulty interpreting the perspectives of others and so Social Stories™ are designed to provide an understanding of the social context for a given situation. Social Stories™ are not a panacea as a social pragmatic intervention; rather they are designed for specific social contexts. Therefore, an autistic student may benefit from exposure to multiple stories to address different social situations. For example, an autistic student may have a social story targeting school arrival routines and a second social story addressing interactions with peers in the playground.

Gray and colleagues (Gray, 2010; Gray & Garand, 1993) delineated several suggestions for developing Social Stories™. For example, practitioners who develop the social story (e.g., the teacher or clinician) should consider the perspective of the autistic child in the context of a specific social situation. In other words, every social story should be individualized to meet the needs of that child in that context. In addition, the mode of delivery of the social story should be tailored to the child's ability level. For example, a social story may consist of simple written sentences tailored to the reading level of the child. Alternatively, a social story may consist of pictures or video vignettes for children who cannot read. The social story is then practiced with the child prior to the targeted social situation. For example, the teacher may read the social story with the student at the beginning of the school day or immediately prior to the social situation targeted in the story (e.g., prior to recess where the student will practice social skills with peers). Additionally, the student may have access to the social story throughout the school day so that he or she can consult the story as needed or practice with the teacher. The child's comprehension of the story should be assessed following story practice. Comprehension can be tested by asking the child to recall the basic tenets of the story. For children with more severe language impairment, comprehension could be tested via roleplay. Essentially, Social Story™ construction and mode of delivery are quite flexible.

In terms of content, a social story usually consists of short basic concepts/phrases that are tailored to the child's comprehension level. Concepts are described as *descriptive*, *directive*, and *perspective*. Descriptive concepts are critical to all social stories, and these describe who the actors are in a social situation and what they do. Descriptive concepts *"paint the social backdrop"* (Gray & Garand, 1993, p. 3) of the story. Each descriptive concept should be presented individually and delivered via an accessible medium to the student, such as written as a sentence on a piece of paper or as an individualized video vignette. A social story may consist entirely of descriptive concepts if the student can independently generate appropriate social responses for that social situation. If it is difficult for the student to independently generate appropriate responses, then a directive concept can be included. A directive concept will describe the appropriate responses for that context. Again, directive responses will be delivered individually via an accessible medium (e.g., the student might view a video vignette of a model roleplaying the appropriate social skills). Finally, perspective concepts may be included in the story. Perspective concepts describe consequences or reactions to the social situation contingent on successful performance of the social skills. For example, the fact that a parent or teacher will be grateful and happy when the student completes a particular task.

In an important early intervention study, Kuttler et al. (1998) examined the use of Social Stories™ to address the problem behavior of a 12-year-old boy with autism and Fragile X syndrome. His communication scores ranged from 2 to 5 years per formal testing. He used one- or two-word utterances that were difficult to understand. He had some manual signs, gestures, and used a communication book that contained 100 symbols. The student attended a self-contained classroom of a residential school with seven other students of similar diagnoses. He exhibited frequent tantrums across the day, particularly during unexpected transitions, wait time, and unstructured free times. A variety of interventions including picture schedule and token system had failed to adequately reduce his tantrums.

A social story was developed for two of the most problematic periods (when tantrums occurred most frequently) of the school day (i.e., lunch and work). The social stories were developed according to guidelines outlined by Gray and Garand (1993) and consisted of five and seven concepts for work and lunch, respectively. Each social story was presented in an individual booklet with a concept on each page that was presented simultaneously in print and as an icon. For example, the work social story was presented on five individual pages, which included the concept in print plus an icon depicting the concept. The print sentences on each individual page for the work social story are presented in Table 10.2.

The stories were read to the student by the teaching staff immediately prior to work and lunch periods. The student had access to the booklets during lunch and work and was asked by staff to refer to the story when a tantrum precursor occurred. The effects of the social stories were evaluated using an ABAB reversal design, replicated across lunch and work periods. The results showed an almost complete elimination of precursor tantrum behaviors when social stories were in use in both settings. When social stories were removed, precursor tantrum behaviors returned to similar levels that were evident prior to introducing the intervention in both settings. While this research by Kuttler et al. (1998) was conducted with only a single student, the results suggest that this type of social story intervention may be promising for addressing tantrums, which are not uncommon in children with autism.

Another example of a Social Stories™ evaluation using a single-case experimental design was conducted by Chan and O'Reilly (2008). This study involved two boys (aged 5 and 6 years) who attended two separate kindergarten classrooms in a public elementary school. Both children were diagnosed as autistic and experienced language delays. Both children attended fully inclusive kindergarten classrooms, and the intervention was evaluated as part of the ongoing classroom routine. This appears to be the first published study to examine the effectiveness of a social story intervention within inclusive regular classroom settings. Three behaviors were targeted for each of the students (e.g., inappropriate social interactions, inappropriate, vocalizations, appropriate social initiation).

A total of three stories were developed for each student reflecting each of their three target behaviors. The social stories were developed in accordance with suggested guidelines (Gray & Garand, 1993). Students practiced the social stories at the beginning of the school day by reading them aloud with the help of an instructor. Students then answered comprehension questions about the stories and stories were repeated if students were unable to answer the questions. Finally, students role-played the social situation with the instructor and a confederate and received positive feedback and prompts as necessary.

Table 10.2 Printed sentences for the work social story used by Kuttler et al. (1998)

Page	Sentence
1	We do work time at school every day.
2	When Nancy picks me up in the mornings, I need to wait nicely at the door.
3	When I finish my work with Nancy, she gives me a sticker.
4	When I come back to class for circle time, I get another sticker.
5	I like to earn stickers; I can pick a prize.

Student behaviors were measured in their regular kindergarten classrooms during circle time and center time on the same day as training sessions. The effectiveness of the social story intervention was assessed using a multiple baseline across behaviors design. Hence, social story training was sequentially staggered across each of the three target skills for each participant. Results of the social stories intervention demonstrated a clear effect with decreases in inappropriate behavior (e.g., inappropriate vocalizations) and increases in appropriate behaviors (e.g., appropriate social interactions) when the intervention was applied. Additionally, positive effects were evident for up to 10 months post intervention. The skills also generalized to a new school year with a different classroom and teacher.

Visual Activity Schedules

A visual activity schedule (VAS) is another form of visual support that has been used in an effort to promote completion and understanding of routines and social situations for persons with severe disabilities who have limited or no speech. VAS have consisted of a set of pictorial cues that are provided prior to an activity or series of activities and that aim to support the person to successfully navigate the activities. These visual cues typically illustrate a sequence of tasks or activities, which may guide the person through the routines, tasks, or activities. In some respects, VAS are similar to Social Stories™ in that they could be conceptualized as representing a set of antecedent cues to enhance understanding of social context and prompt successful performance. In practice, however, VAS tend to focus on successful performance of a multistep task sequence across an entire school day, whereas Social Stories™ tend to focus on guiding the person's social and emotional reactions to specific social situations.

VAS are popular in clinical and educational settings and are often used to facilitate the performance of activities that may be difficult for the person to recall, initiate, and/or complete. VAS are also used to signal transitions between tasks, supplement verbal directions, and reduce problem behavior when transitioning from preferred to nonpreferred activities. They are often used as part of a broader package of instructional supports that include systematic instructional procedures (e.g., time delay, least-to-most prompting, reinforcement) to facilitate and strengthen correct responding. Visual supports have long been championed as important components of comprehensive support strategies for individuals with severe disabilities who have limited or no speech. For example, Brown (1991) recommended that visual activity schedules be considered when managing problem behavior as part of an overall positive behavior support system. Additionally, Mesibov et al. (2002) described VAS as a critical component of the TEACCH model, which is a comprehensive educational system designed specifically to support the needs of school children with autism. Individuals with severe disabilities, such as autism, may fail to attend and respond to salient cues during instruction. Additionally, autistic individuals are often described as visual learners who may experience difficulties with auditory processing and executive functioning (Fleury et al., 2014). Hence, visual schedules might help with organizing, sequencing, and planning activities. Combining visual supports with verbal instructions may enhance understanding of expectations and routines, thereby facilitating skill acquisition and minimizing the impact of problem behaviors.

VAS often consist of a series of laminated pictures, photographs, or symbols that represent key activities over the course of a given period of the day, such as activities across a morning school routine (e.g., circle time, reading, play, quiet time). Pictures representing each activity can be individually attached in the sequence in which the activities will occur on a sentence strip and placed in a visible area of the classroom or may be attached to individual pages of a booklet that the student carries with them across class routines. The visual cues representing different activities of a VAS are selected based on the abilities of the student. For students with visual impairment, the use of tangible symbols to represent each activity may be indicated (e.g., a small toy representing a play period). A VAS using tangible symbols (see Chap. 6) could be presented with individual items representing a given activity in individual boxes or on individual shelves. The sequence of activities is typically presented in a top to bottom or from left to right sequence. An example of a VAS is presented in Fig. 10.1.

VAS instruction might begin by teaching the student to associate each activity (e.g., playtime) with a given picture or tangible symbol (e.g., a laminated picture of a toy or small physical toy). The student is simultaneously taught to sequence the visual cues to reflect the order in which each activity will occur as part of the classroom routine, for example. As the routine progresses through the day, the student is taught to return to the schedule, indicate the end of one activity (e.g., by removing the laminated picture of that activity from the sentence strip and placing it in a container beside the VAS), and then initiate the next activity that is displayed on the VAS. The teacher might need to prompt and verbally describe the end of one activity and the beginning of the next activity as the student updates the VAS. Students may receive positive consequences for using the VAS correctly. For example, a student may receive a token for accurately using the VAS to transition from one activity to the next activity. Tokens can then be exchanged at the end of the school day for preferred items. Students might also be involved in selecting the sequence of activities at the beginning of a school day. They may also be given opportunities to choose between tasks or materials (e.g., using paints versus drawing pens) during an activity. Incorporating a student's preferences and choices within the VAS may be one

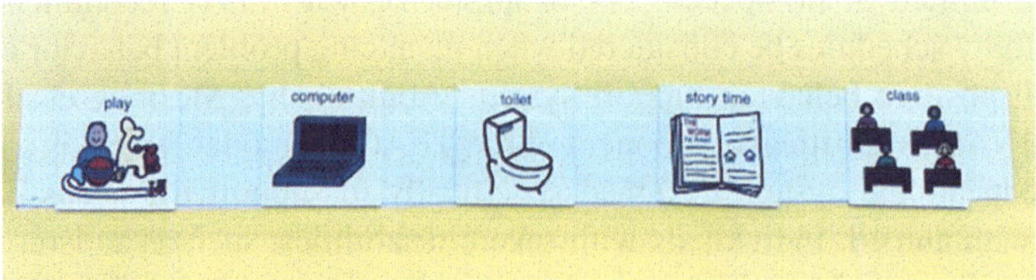

Fig. 10.1 Example of a visual activity schedule for a classroom routine

way to support self-determination and reduce the possibility of transition-related problem behavior (Lequia et al., 2011). Similar instructional strategies can be used to implement VAS in other contexts, such as the home.

VAS have been examined to enhance early play skills for children with severe disabilities. The development of early play skills is foundational to establishing and enhancing children's communication and social skills and may also help decrease problem behaviors such as aggression, tantrums, and self-injury (Thorp et al., 1995).

Morrison et al. (2002) examined the use of VAS to teach play skills to four autistic preschoolers in an inclusive classroom setting. The children's ages ranged between 42 and 70 months at the time of the study. All four children were diagnosed with autism and exhibited significant deficits in receptive and expressive language development. Three of the children did not speak. Eight typically developing same-aged peers attended the classroom. The classroom was divided into four play areas: Blocks, Kitchen, Dollhouse, and Art. Age-appropriate toys designed to facilitate interactive play were available in each play area.

A VAS was implemented with each of the autistic children to facilitate on-task play behavior and play correspondence. Prior to playtime, the children were individually presented with four photographs of each of the play areas and were asked by the instructor, *Where do you want to play?* The children were prompted to select one photograph and attach it to a clipboard. Each child was prompted to select three play areas and attached the three corresponding photographs to their clipboard from left to right. Children were then prompted to *Follow your play schedule*. An enlarged photograph (same as the photograph on the child's clipboard) was displayed at each play area. The child was to attend each play area in the sequence selected on their clipboard. The child received least-to-most prompts (verbal to physical) from an instructor to follow the play schedule and to appropriately play with toys if they were off-task or engaged in stereotypic behavior.

Each child's on-task behavior (e.g., appropriately engaging with toys and verbal and nonverbal interactions with other students), off-task behavior (e.g., mouthing, finger flicking, bouncing, spinning), disruptive behavior (e.g., aggression), and the correspondence between the child's picture schedule and use of play areas were measured. The effects of the picture activity schedule (plus instructor prompts) were evaluated using a multiple baseline across participants' design. Each of the four children showed an increase with respect to on-task behavior, peer interactions, and correspondence between the photographic schedule and play areas chosen when the intervention was introduced. Decreases in problem behavior were also evident. Overall, the results from Morrison et al. (2002) indicate that the VAS plus instructor prompting procedure successfully taught the children to navigate these important play settings and acted as a nonintrusive strategy to foster important communication and social skills.

In another example, Krantz et al. (1993) taught three families to implement a photographic schedule with their autistic children in the home. Parents often report difficulties managing these children's problem behaviors and skills deficits and this situation can impede routine family activities and functioning. Three children, aged 6, 7, and 8 years, participated. All were diagnosed with autism and received overall adaptive age equivalency scores of about 2 years. Children were taught to use a VAS in a clinical setting, which was then generalized to the home. Each child was given a three-ring binder with a photograph on each page. Children were taught to open the binder, point to the first photograph, engage in the task represented by that photograph, return to the binder, and turn the page for the next activity. An instructor used graduate guidance to prompt following of the photographic schedule.

The VAS was then implemented in the home setting, and parents were taught to manage their child's use of the photographic schedule. The schedule was implemented for about 4 hours each afternoon (between school ending and dinner time) and individualized activities were incorporated into the photographic schedule to suit the family (e.g., hanging up a coat, putting away lunch box, and making a snack). The effects of the VAS were evaluated using a multiple baseline across families' design. Researchers measured engagement (e.g., performing the tasks depicted in the schedule), problem behavior (e.g., tantrums, aggression, and stereotypy), and social initiations (e.g., sharing objects/activities, pointing to or reaching for an object, and verbalizing words).

Overall, the results demonstrated reductions in problem behavior and corresponding increases in engagement and social initiations when the VAS was introduced to each of the families. These positive results maintained for up to 10 months with two families. Parents reported adapting the schedule to successfully include out-of-home activities, such as trips to restaurants.

Indications for Using Visual Strategies for Receptive Communication

The three intervention strategies described in this chapter (augmented input, Social Stories™, and VAS) have produced promising results in terms of improving receptive communication skills among people learners with severe disabilities and significant communication difficulties. Augmented input, including ALM procedures, appears to be a relatively easy strategy to implement in applied settings such as the home or school. Augmented input involves the communication partner utilizing the communication device (e.g., pointing to pictures on the communication board or SGD) while simultaneously speaking to the student. Augmented input has been demonstrated to increase receptive vocabulary and research demonstrates that ALM can be successfully implemented in regular family contexts. It may be beneficial if researchers and therapists combined expressive and receptive communication strategies simultaneously when developing interventions for nonverbal and minimally verbal people with severe disabilities.

Social Stories™ can be seen as representing a social problem-solving approach for improving adaptive-social functioning. These stories are relatively simple to develop and include a description of the social rules and actors in a social situation coupled with suggestions for how to behave or react in that context. The story is tailored to the student needs and can include written instructions and/or pictures. The teacher or parent can walk the learner through these rules and roleplay the social skills. Social Stories™ could be seen as a type of antecedent self-regulation intervention. The specific instructional approach used in teaching the person to respond to a social story typically incorporates many behavior-analytic principles and procedures (e.g., response prompting, prompt fading, and reinforcement). Research evaluations have generally found these types of antecedent interventions and systematic instructional tactics to be successful for teaching communication, social, and other adaptive skills to people with severe disabilities.

VAS are used extensively in educational and clinical settings and have been evaluated by researchers. VAS serve as a series of visual antecedent cues that can consist of items, pictures, or symbols that will signal the sequence and nature of upcoming activities. A VAS can be placed in a prominent area of a classroom or home, or it could be carried by the learner in a booklet. The learner is taught to navigate the VAS through a series of prompts and use of reinforcement delivered by the teacher or parent. VAS have been shown to increase adaptive responding, facilitate choice-making, and reduce problem behavior. VAS may work in part by helping facilitate an understanding of the overall structure of routines.

Contraindications for Using Visual Strategies for Receptive Communication

A variety of strategies of augmented input have been suggested in the literature (e.g., ALM and ALS). However, research to support the use of such strategies in applied settings is relatively limited. Additionally, there seems to be a proliferation of nomenclature essentially describing what appears to be similar sets of strategies, that is, the communication partner's use of aided AAC to provide supplemental input during communication interactions. Further research is needed to document the efficacy of augmented input with aided AAC to enhance receptive communication skills. For instance, research to date has focused on comprehension of individual words and not so much on the development of syntax. Additionally, the development of user-friendly measures of receptive communication might help applied researchers, clinicians, and educators to document change during augmented input interventions.

While Social Stories™ are popular and widely used in educational settings, the mechanisms that affect change in social behavior are not clearly understood. Successful implementation of Social Stories™ may depend in part on how well teachers and others provide instruction, create practice opportunities via roleplay opportunities, prompt appropriate social responses, and arrange reinforcing consequences for appropriate responding. Component analyses of Social Stories™ may be warranted to tease out the effective or critical elements of what is in effect a multicomponent intervention. Nevertheless, Social Stories™ interventions are popular and are generally supported as effective by the research literature.

VAS have been extensively researched in educational and home contexts and are ubiquitous in classrooms and other settings supporting individuals with severe disabilities with limited communication skills. Successful implementation of VAS may require upskilling parents and educators in the use of certain instructional strategies, such as prompting and reinforcement procedures, preference assessment and choice-making protocols, as well as techniques for managing problem behavior. VAS might best be conceived as dynamic antecedent strategies that will likely require input to reflect changes in schedules and should routinely involve the learner as an active participant who is enabled to make choices (when appropriate). Failure to use VAS in a dynamic manner may eventually be counterproductive, serving to reinforce a rigid pattern of activities for the learner, which may lead to escalation of problem behavior when routines or choices cannot be honored.

Implementation Considerations

Three sets of aided AAC strategies to enhance receptive communication for persons with severe communication delays have been described in this chapter (i.e., augmented input techniques, Social Stories™, and VAS). Each of these strategies is designed to enhance various aspects of receptive communication, including understanding vocabulary. Augmented input such as ALM is a relatively friendly set of techniques that seem to be relatively easy to implement by a parent or educator. ALM involves pointing to the targeted items and activities in the environment and to the pictures on the device while vocalizing the word. ALM could conceivably be included as part of a comprehensive instructional approach, which could also involve teaching requesting skills, for example. A set of targeted receptive vocabulary would need to be identified prior to intervention and parents or teachers would need to be taught how to use augmented input. Reliable methods that will provide a valid assessment of receptive communication are complicated and can be difficult to implement in applied settings, which complicates the evaluation of intervention efficacy.

Social Stories™ have mainly focused on teaching social interaction/social communication skills. The targeted social situation should be described in a simple and accessible format for the learner (using words or pictures or a combination as appropriate). Appropriate responses within the targeted social situations should also be presented in a similar accessible format. The story should be practiced prior to the targeted social situation. This practice may involve presentation of the story, modeling and roleplay of targeted social behaviors, and reinforcement for appropriate responding by the learner during roleplay. Presentation and practice of the social story can be brief and can be conducted with the learner on a one-to-one basis. Performance of the targeted social skills should be assessed in the real-world setting and assessment results used to decide whether the intervention needs to be modified. Social Stories™ seem to be relatively easy to implement, and data show that such interventions can produce positive results.

VAS are common in clinical and educational settings. Research has demonstrated that VAS can enhance independence, enable choice-making, and reduce problem behavior. The visual display chosen should reflect the ability level of the learner and could make use of tangible symbols, line drawing, photographs of activities, or a combination of such communication symbols. The visual display should be presented in a manner that is accessible to the student, such as in a picture book or with individual pictures presented on a sentence strip. The learner is taught to follow the pictorial sequence and can be actively involved in using the VAS to navigate through the sequence of routines (e.g., removing the picture of an activity once completed and identifying the next activity). Where possible, the student should be encouraged to make choices between activities. New activities should be introduced to the routine periodically to extend the person's range of activities, develop greater independence, and maintain the person's interest in participating in activities and in using and following visual schedules. Incorporating choice and changes in activities as part of the VAS may promote independence and self-determination and might also reduce problem behavior when, on occasion, the anticipated routine cannot be honored. Materials used to develop a VAS are accessible and inexpensive. However, successfully implementing a VAS requires knowledge of systematic instructional strategies (e.g., response prompting, prompt fading, and reinforcement). Competencies related to the provision for choice and management of problem behavior are also likely to be relevant for many people with severe disabilities involved in a VAS intervention.

Summary and Conclusion

The use of visual strategies to support successful receptive communication for non-verbal and minimally verbal people with severe disabilities was addressed in this chapter. Receptive communication can be defined as a person's ability to understand vocabulary, syntax, and pragmatics. Three visual intervention strategies designed to support receptive communication were described (i.e., augmented input, Social Stories™, and VAS). Key studies evaluating the use of these three strategies provide empirical support for their use to improve receptive communication.

Augmented input includes a series of strategies used with aided AAC devices to support receptive vocabulary and syntax. Augmented input strategies such as ALM are fairly simple to implement and appear to increase single-word use. But research on the use of augmented input to support receptive communication with this population is limited and there is a need for more research into the value of augmented input to enhance areas such as syntax development. Both Social Stories™ and VAS are popular strategies in clinical and educational settings. They involve, among other things, verbal and visual cues to help the person navigate social interactions and follow a schedule of daily routines, respectively. There is a solid research base to support the use of Social Stories™ and VAS in applied settings. While the materials used to construct Social Stories™ and VAS are inexpensive and easily accessible, successful implementation of these strategies requires competencies in using systematic instructional strategies.

References

Allen, A. A., Schlosser, R. W., Brock, K. L., & Shane, H. C. (2017). The effectiveness of aided augmented input techniques for persons with developmental disabilities: A systematic review. *Augmentative and Alternative Communication, 33*(3), 149–159. https://doi.org/10.1080/07434618.2017.1338752

Arthur-Kelly, M., Sigafoos, J., Green, V., Mathisen, B., & Arthur-Kelly, R. (2009). Issues in the use of visual supports to promote communication in individuals with autism spectrum disorder. *Disability and Rehabilitation, 31*(18), 1474–1486. https://doi.org/10.1080/09638280802590629

Binger, C., & Light, J. (2007). The effect of aided AAC modeling on the expression of multi-symbol messages by preschoolers who use AAC. *Augmentative and Alternative Communication, 23*(1), 30–43. Erratum in *Augmentative and Alternative Communication*, *23*(2), 2007, 188–189. https://doi.org/10.1080/07434610600807470

Brown, F. (1991). Creative daily scheduling: A nonintrusive approach to problem behaviors in community residences. *Journal of the Association for Persons with Severe Handicaps, 16*(2), 75–84. https://doi.org/10.1177/154079699101600201

Chan, J. M., & O'Reilly, M. F. (2008). A Social Stories™ intervention package for students with autism in inclusive classroom settings. *Journal of Applied Behavior Analysis, 41*(3), 405–409. https://doi.org/10.1901/jaba.2008.41-405

Chazin, K. T., Ledford, J. R., & Pak, N. S. (2021). A systematic review of augmented input interventions and exploratory analysis of moderators. *American Journal of Speech and Language Pathology, 30*(3), 1210–1223. https://doi.org/10.1044/2020_AJSLP-20-00102

Crowe, B., Machalicek, W., Wei, Q., Drew, C., & Ganz, J. (2022). Augmentative and alternative communication for children with intellectual and developmental disability: A mega-review of the literature. *Journal of Developmental and Physical Disabilities, 34*(1), 1–42. https://doi.org/10.1007/s10882-021-09790-0

Dada, S., Flores, C., Bastable, K., & Schlosser, R. W. (2021). The effects of augmentative and alternative communication interventions on the receptive language skills of children with developmental disabilities: A scoping review. *International Journal of Speech-Language Pathology, 23*(3), 247–257. https://doi.org/10.1080/17549507.2020.1797165

Douglas, S. N., Meadan, H., Biggs, E. E., Bagawan, A., & Kaori Terol, A. (2023). Building family capacity: Supporting multiple family members to implement aided language modeling. *Journal of Autism and Developmental Disorders, 53*(7), 2587–2599. https://doi.org/10.1007/s10803-022-05492-4

Drager, K. D., Postal, V. J., Carrolus, L., Castellano, M., Gagliano, C., & Glynn, J. (2006). The effect of aided language modelling on symbol comprehension and production in two preschoolers with autism. *American Journal of Speech-Language Pathology, 15*(2), 112–125. https://doi.org/10.1044/1058-0360(2006/012)

Fleury, V. P., Hedges, S., Hume, K., Browder, D., Thompson, J., Fallin, K., El Zein, F., Reutebuch, C., & Vaughn, S. (2014). Addressing the academic needs of adolescents with autism spectrum disorder in secondary education. *Remedial and Special Education, 35*(2), 68–79. https://doi.org/10.1177/0741932513518823

Gray, C. (2010). *The new Social Story™ book*. Future Horizons.

Gray, C., & Garand, J. D. (1993). Social stories: Improving responses of students with autism with accurate social information. *Focus on Autistic Behavior, 8(1)*, 1–10.

Harris, M. D., & Reichle, J. (2004). The impact of aided language stimulation on symbol comprehension and production in children with moderate cognitive disabilities. *American Journal of Speech-Language Pathology, 13*(2), 155–167. https://doi.org/10.1044/1058-0360(2004/016)

Krantz, P. J., Mac Duff, M. T., & McClannahan, L. E. (1993). Programming participation in family activities for children with autism: parents use of photographic activity schedules. *Journal of Applied Behavior Analysis, 26*(*1*), 137–138. https://doi.org/10.1901/jaba.1993.26-137

Kuttler, S., Myles, B. S., & Carlson, J. K. (1998). The use of social stories to reduce precursors to tantrum behavior in a student with autism. *Focus on Autism and Other Developmental Disabilities, 13*(3), 176–182. https://doi.org/10.1177/108835769801300306

Lequia, J., Machalicek, W., & Rispoli, M. (2011). Effects of activity schedules on problem behavior exhibited in children with autism spectrum disorders: A systematic review. *Research in Autism Spectrum Disorders, 6*(1), 480–492. https://doi.org/10.1016/j.rasd.2011.07.008

Mesibov, G. B., Browder, D. M., & Kirkland, C. (2002). Using individualized schedules as a component of positive behavioral support for students with developmental disabilities. *Journal of Positive Behavior Interventions, 4*(2), 73–79. https://doi.org/10.1177/109830070200400202

Morrison, R. S., Sainato, D. M., Benchaaban, D., & Endo, S. (2002). Increasing play skills of children with autism using activity schedules and correspondence training. *Journal of Early Intervention, 25*(1), 58–72. https://doi.org/10.1177/105381510202500106

Romski, M. A., & Sevcik, R. A. (1997). Augmentative and alternative communication for children with developmental disabilities. *Mental Retardation and Developmental Disabilities Research Reviews, 3*(4), 363–368. https://doi.org/10.1002/(SICI)1098-2779(1997)3:4<363::AID-MRDD12>3.0.CO;2-T

Thorp, D. M., Stahmer, A. C., & Schreibman, L. (1995). Effects of sociodramatic play training on children with autism. *Journal of Autism and Developmental Disorders, 25*(3), 265–282. https://doi.org/10.1007/BF02179288

Index

J. Sigafoos et al., *Communication Strategies for People with Severe Disabilities*, Autism and Child Psychopathology Series,
https://doi.org/10.1007/978-3-031-83807-1

The manufacturer's authorised representative in the EU is Springer Nature Customer Service Centre GmbH, Europaplatz 3, 69115 Heidelberg, Germany. If you have any concerns regarding our products, please contact ProductSafety@springernature.com

Printed and bound by CPI Group (UK) Ltd, Croydon, CR0 4YY
30/09/2026
02225600-0001